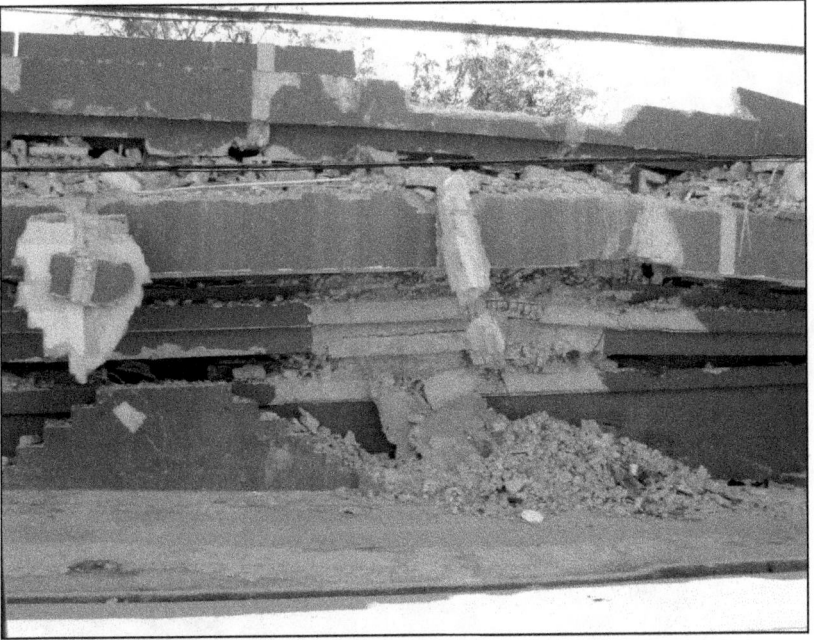

One of the most powerful pictures I have taken in Haiti. Representative of the disaster, this three story building is completely destroyed. Hundreds of bodies lay inside sandwiched between concrete.

*"When one walks with humility in this world, their footsteps are heard in paradise".*

- Anonymous Muslim Scholar -

# Where's Haiti?

*Personal Profiles Of Life After The Devastation*

## Tipu V. Khan, M.D.

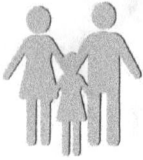

# DOCTIPU

w w w . d o c t i p u . c o m

Doc Tipu, L.L.C.

www.DocTipu.com

Copyright © 2013 by Tipu Khan

First published February 2013

Library of Congress Control Number: 2013900504

ISBN (paperback black & white images) 978-0-9888576-1-2

ISBN (paperback color images) 978-0-9888576-2-9

ISBN (Ebook) 978-0-9888576-0-5

Edited by Susie Medina

www.TheFilmChild.com

Cover Art and Interior Design: Ali Majoka
http://www.facebook.com/grafikali.seven

THE AUTHOR IS DONATING A LARGE PORTION OF HIS NET PROCEEDS FROM THIS BOOK TO NON-PROFIT MEDICAL ORGANIZATIONS WORKING IN HAITI AND ELSEWHERE AROUND THE WORLD

*To my family – without you, none of this would be possible.*

*To Hamza – the world is yours, and so am I.*

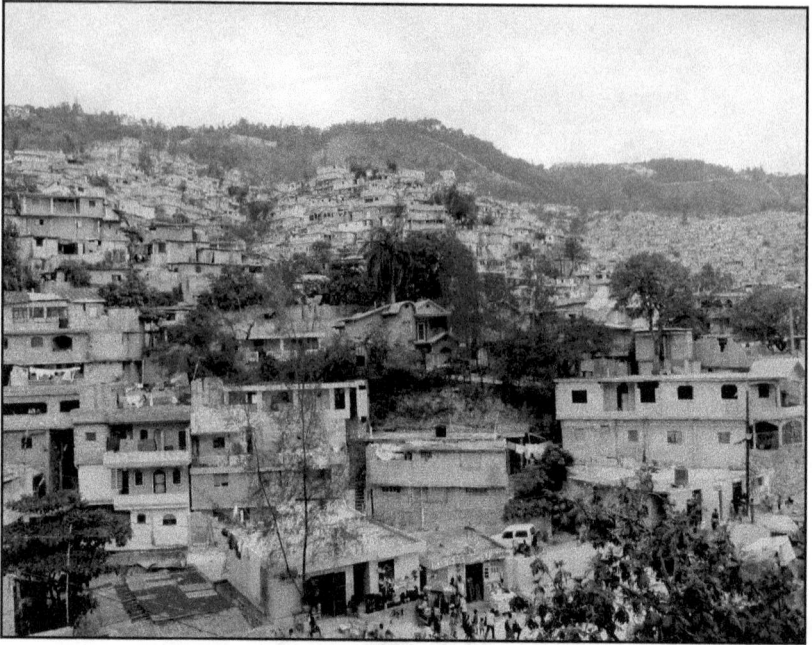

Areas of PaP have some of the most poverty dense housing in the Western Hemisphere. This made search and rescue nearly impossible in certain neighborhoods.

*...Haiti is one place where humans are increasingly endangered.*

- Dr. Varun Verma, Undo Inaction, 2011 -

# Contents

Acronyms and Abbreviations

Preface                                    1

Introduction                               8

Where's Haiti?                            24

The Aftermath                             32

Bienvenue à Haïti!                        42

The Loa                                   58

Common Things Being Common                76

Balrog                                    98

Night Sweats                             110

Dance of the Mind                        132

Kissing Emily                            152

Life Goes On                             178

Taking Care of Ourselves                 198

Closing Thoughts                         220

Acknowledgments                          226

# Acronyms and Abbreviations

AIDS – Acquired Immune Deficiency Syndrome

CT – Computed Tomography

ECG – Electrocardiogram

EEG – Electroencephologram

ER – Emergency Room

FEMA – Federal Emergency Management Agency

FM – Family Medicine

GI - Gastrointestinal

HBMPM – Hospital Bernard Mevs Project Medishare

HIV – Human Immune Deficiency Virus

ICU – Intensive Care Unit

IV - Intravenous

MDR TB – Multidrug Resistant Tuberculosis

MSF – Medecins Sans Frontiers

NGO – Non Governmental Organization

NPO – Non Profit Organization

PaP – Port-Au-Prince

PNH - Police Nationale d'Haïti

PM – Project Medishare

OB – Obstetrics

OR – Operating Room

RSI – Rapid Sequence Intubation

TB – Tuberculosis

UN – United Nations

US – United States

USD – United States Dollars

WHO – World Health Organization

WMD – Weapons of Mass Destruction

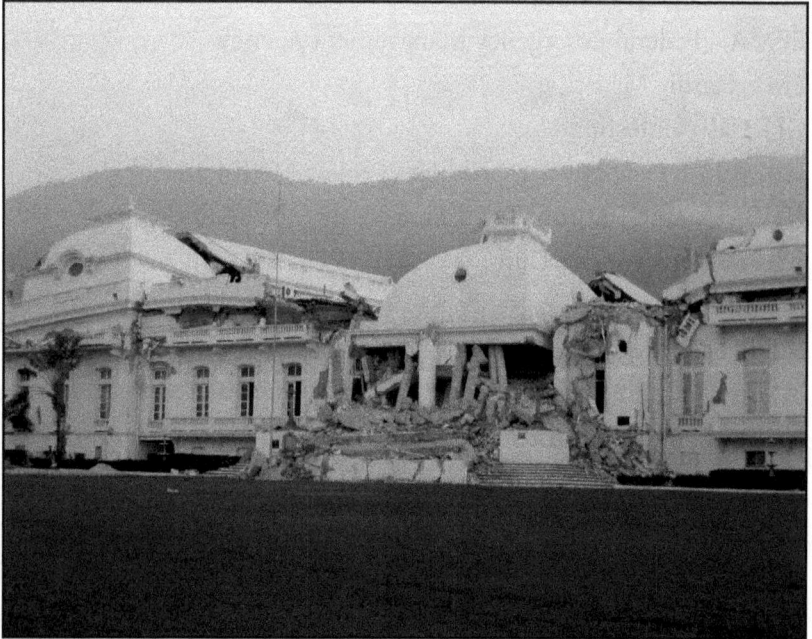

Haiti's Capital Building.

# Preface

What does it mean to be a doctor? The word doctor comes from the Latin word *docēre*, which means 'to teach.' In the past, the term was used loosely in association with anyone in a formal teaching position. Church Apostles, school teachers, and physicians were all doctors. As higher education became more formalized the word doctor became more specific – signifying some level of higher mastery and formal education such as law, medicine, or theology. A doctor during this time was an expert on medicine, theology, and more. This was the time of the true Renaissance Man. Later, those who pursued higher education in clinical medical practice were given the title of *Doctor of Medicine* or M.D. (Medicinae Doctor).

A doctor has been formally educated and received the highest degree in the practice of medicine. After completing a four year bachelor's degree in college we go on to complete a four year medical degree in medical school. After medical school, we choose a specialty and complete residency training that can last anywhere from three to seven years. Some of us go on to sub-specialize or sub-sub-specialize which can be another one to four years. Keeping count yet? That's 11 years at minimum and up to 15 years plus after graduating high school. By the time a doctor has completed training they are typically between 29 to 33 years old at minimum. Sometimes we even go back and retrain in another specialty, adding an additional 3+ years to that age.

During training we are paid a tad over minimum wage working

an average anywhere from 60-90+ hours a week. That gives us just enough money to survive but not enough to work on chiseling away at our debt. According to the American Medical Association in 2011 86-91% of graduating medical students complete school with $162,000 to $205,674 of educational debt. When adjusted for inflation from 1978 the debt has more than tripled! While friends who graduated high school with me are buying cars, homes, and having kids we're starting our professional career with a debt equivalent to a mortgage on our credit. Delayed gratification is a way of life for physicians. We put in the work now and expect some payback in years to come. Most of us don't pay off our educational debt until we hit the age of 50. $200,000 with interest paid over 20 years amounts to over $400,000 in most cases and up $600,000 in some. When we start off in our field our credit score is poor (high debt to low income ratio). This makes buying a house or even a car very difficult for a doctor at the age of 32. So we're not really financially secure until we hit our mid 40's.

With an educational loan higher than many people's mortgage it is no wonder why many bright and capable prospects from poverty backgrounds do not pursue a career in medicine. Those that do are burdened with debt for 20-30 years of their career. Many choose higher paying specialties for financial reasons – creating a paucity of primary care physicians who have traditionally been paid less than the specialist. Without a guide to emphasize primary care and prevention, more and more Americans are getting sick. We are having complications of diabetes and hypertension that aren't seen as frequently in countries where primary care is emphasized such as The United Kingdom, Japan, and Canada. With high amounts of debt it is increasingly hard to convince doctors to *prevent* an ailment when they can get paid more to *fix* an ailment!

That is a crash course on how to *become* a doctor and *what* a doctor is but what does it really mean *to be* a doctor? The doctor is a healer, a clinician. Overtly our job is simple – to heal. Healing, though, is a complex idea with many facets. For a human to heal we need nurturing on various levels. Sometimes we need medications to cure an ailment, sometimes rest, and other times mental support and confidence to overcome trying times. The body is a complex machine and sometimes it can be healed and at other times it cannot.

For doctors to be able to heal patients we need certain tools. We have fancy machines and tools by which we diagnose an ailment. We are granted the ability to access formulated compounds and drugs which cause lasting and sometimes irreversible changes in the human body. These changes are mostly for the good but can occasionally be for the worse. Every drug, every treatment, every intervention has its side effects. We weigh the risks of a treatment to the benefit and when the benefits significantly outweigh the risks, we provide said treatment. Sometimes the adverse effect of a treatment is high but this is a chance we calculate and an outcome we are ready to accept. This level of responsibility over the human body is what we are trained to accept.

Healing the human body and spirit requires us to get to know our patients and their social situations well. When poverty requires a diabetic to eat processed fast food twice a day because it is substantially cheaper than purchasing fresh fruits and vegetables, prescribing a pill will not have its full intended effect. When the leading cause of death in adolescents and young adults in the U.S. is violence and car accidents, what good does it do if I constantly harp on healthy eating or safe sex? We are just trying to play catch up instead of treating the true barriers to healthy living in our patients. How can doctors provide better food choices to a poor diabetic or lower the rates of gang violence? Social and political activism.

Doctors hold a unique position in society. We are trained healers who can identify the barriers to care and healthy living in society. Many of these barriers are not of a biological medical cause, but rather a social or political one. Thus it is only natural that doctors find themselves as social and political advocates for their patients' wellbeing. We write letters to our congressmen, author bills for the senate, run for public office, and sit on city councils and housing authority boards. We fight big corporations who do not provide reasonable living salaries and benefits for employees. Doctors boycott companies that contribute to childhood obesity. We refuse to purchase items from organizations that do business with countries that routinely practice genocide and apartheid even in this day and age. We go to war to protect our soldiers who are protecting us. Doctors hold a substantial amount of social and political prowess in society and work hard to use it to better our patients' livelihood.

In its simplest form a doctor is a glorified mechanic who maintains the human body and fixes it when it is broken. What does it mean to me *to be* a doctor? A doctor is a person whose goal is to advance society politically, ethically, humanistically, and medically. A doctor is a social and political leader; an advocate for the voices of those who can't be heard. A soldier for those fighting the war against poverty. Above all a doctor is a person. A father, a brother, a mother, sister, daughter, lover, and a human. A doctor bleeds and a doctor hurts but continues to fight on for society.

In this book a doctor will journey through a country devastated by poverty, famine, and natural disasters while challenging the readers understanding of humanity, empathy, grief and love. He will emerge ready to educate and better the world one life at a time – starting with the patients he sees and ending with you, the reader.

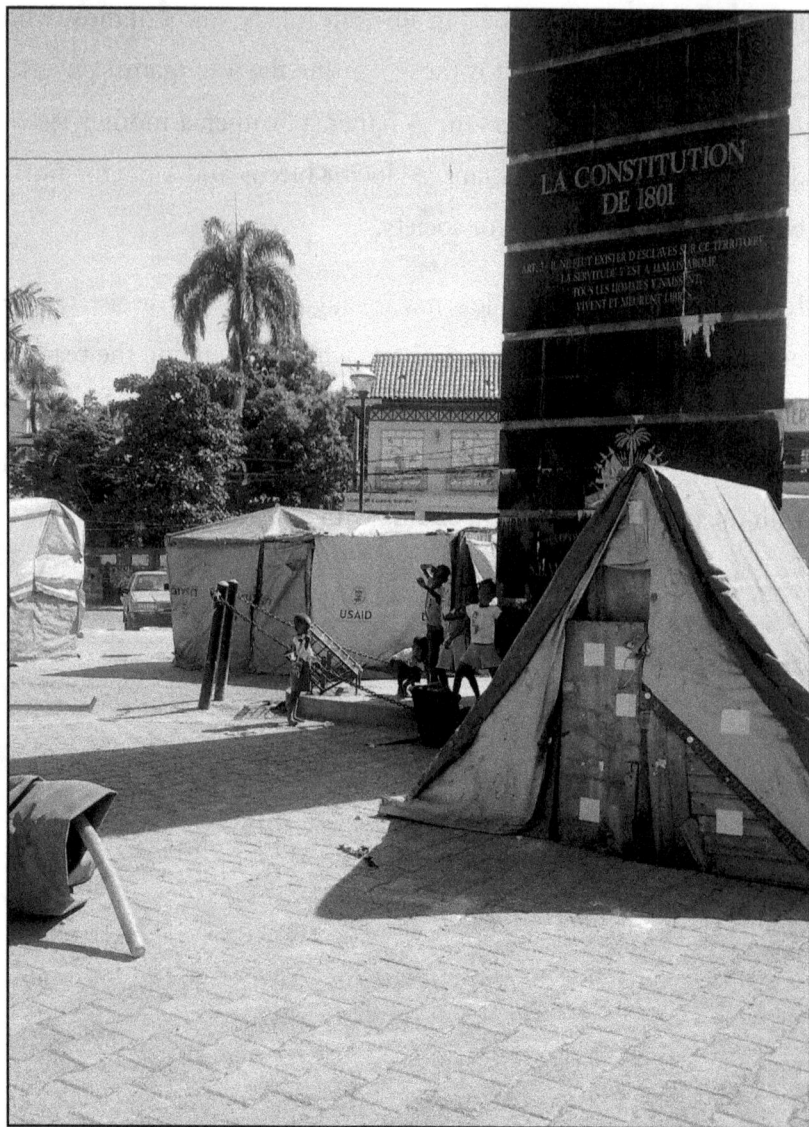

One of the many tent cities. This one at the city center.

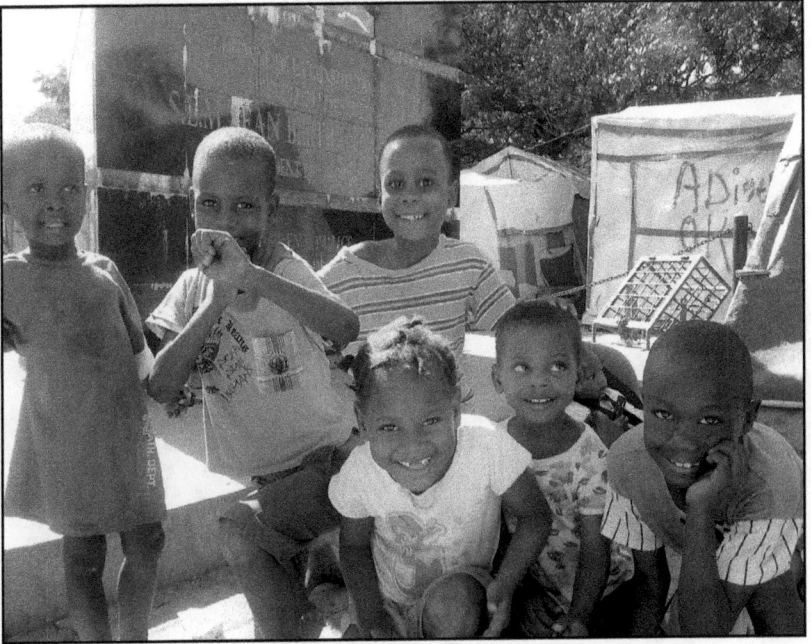

Children living and playing in the city center tent city.

# Introduction

*Act that your principle of action might safely be made a law for the whole world.*

- Immanuel Kant -

Where's Haiti? Can you point it out on a map without looking at the name? How about Haitian history? Did you know what they ate or how they lived? What they found happiness in and how hard they worked for it? Did you hear of the stories of the brave Haitians declaring independence from the French – the first independent slave colony? Had you heard of the thousands of orphans living in Haiti? The HIV epidemic? TB? Paul Farmer? Did you know Haiti? Prior to January 12th, 2010 most of us did not – but now we do.

This book aims to introduce the reader to the ongoing humanitarian crisis which afflicts Haiti. Like most people prior to the earthquake, I had heard of Haiti but was not familiar with its culture or history, the problems they are facing, nor was I even able to point the country out on a map. I didn't know where Haiti was let alone who she was. That all changed as I found myself travelling to the Caribbean after the disaster. My life would never be the same now that I had discovered our neighbor.

Through numerous short stories gathered from multiple humanitarian trips, I will share personal stories and experiences. We will walk through the current humanitarian crisis as most of us have experienced it: with our first real concept of Haiti having formed at the time of the devastating January earthquake. We will start our journey on January 12th, 2010 and continue on though the present.

# Leaving

Sitting in the Orange County, California airport waiting for my flight to Miami, I look outside and know how much I will miss home. The clear blue skies, the cleanliness and amenities, the friends and family, and most of all, my wife. Her sweet caressing touch and caring voice would be so far. In all our years of marriage, we hadn't spent more than a call night or two away from each other. This would prove to be the hardest challenge for me.

My wife and I met in college. I was a peer advisor and she an incoming freshmen. We met to discuss her schedule and that was about it for some time. Interested in me, she began attending some of the club meetings for our major which I was running. We shared some superficial conversations – we chatted about the language of Arabic, school, family, but didn't get far for a few weeks. Knowing I was trying to learn Arabic, she gave me her phone number and email and told me to contact her and she would tutor me. I didn't call her.

A few weeks went by and I hadn't gotten the hint from her yet. So the next time we met, she once again gave me her contact information and told me to get in touch with her. I thought, *when I need help with Arabic, I'll get in touch with her.* I saw her a few more times and learned later that at one point I sat down at her table in the library with friends and we were being fairly loud while studying and forced her to get up and leave the table. I didn't even know she was sitting there. At one point, she even brought me a platter of baklawa she had made (a sweet flaky pastry made throughout the Mediterranean – from Greece to Jordan). I thought nothing of it. People often baked cookies or other treats and brought them in to share. I had no idea how much time went into making the treat. I ate a couple of pieces and shared the rest with my study buddies.

I was a pretty goal oriented college kid at the time. I was the peer advisor for our major, worked 25 hours a week driving busses (UC Davis Unitrans is a student run bus service serving Davis), was in a lab doing research, tutoring, and was practicing Brazilian Jiu-Jitsu four times a week. Any free time I had was spent studying for medical school tests then applying for medical schools followed by interviewing for medical schools. I was busy, to the say the least. The last thing on my radar was taking subtle hints from an interested freshman. I was oblivious.

I've always been good at multi-tasking. I perform better when I have numerous projects on my plate. My father, for example, prefers to complete projects one at a time. I, however, at any given time had at least 3 major projects going on. Even today, when sitting down to watch a movie I will have my laptop open working on some project. I call it functional Attention Deficit Disorder (an oxymoron because part of the definition of A.D.D. is not being able to function normally). Whatever it was, it worked well for me.

About two months into the quarter she was frustrated and had finally had it with me. I was outside the Life Sciences building on campus around noon tabling for our major at an information session when she came up to me. It was already a warm Davis day with a high pollen count by noon. My allergies were held at bay but I was sweating from the sun beating down on me. She walked up to me after I finished with another student and before I could say hi, the verbal onslaught began. She yelled at me. *Why haven't you called me? Why haven't you emailed me? I gave you my number a long time ago and you still haven't called.* It kept going and going. I felt the beads of sweat drip down my brow and the nape of my neck. I hadn't been yelled at like that by any female except my mom. After she finished her rant she retracted her claws and stormed away.

I stood there frozen in place. *What the heck just happened?* I thought. Like my mother likes to say, I was a tube light that day. The switch had been turned on a while ago but the light just flickered on. She was interested in me. All of a sudden it came together. Why hadn't I seen this coming? Why hadn't I acted on this before? She was young, pretty, intelligent, and sweet – what was wrong with me?

The next two hours were spent replaying all our past meetings. The more and more I thought about it, the more I realized how sweet she was: from offering her time to tutor me in Arabic, to chit chatting about family and life, to baking me goodies. A couple hours later I called her and asked her out to dinner. A bit over a year later we were wed. We married young and spent most of our years of education together. We were best friends who studied together, went out together, and spent all our time together. Her friends were mine and mine hers. Our friends joked that they could never get us away from one another. She was, and is, literally the other half of me.

As I sat in the airport, knowing this would be the longest amount of time we were away from each other was very difficult. I sat there at the concourse looking outside at the jets as they took off and landed, eating one of her famous molasses cookies. In a parallel universe I exist as the Cookie Monster. I can't do without a daily quota of cookies. No matter what happened, she wouldn't let me leave the house without a couple of cookies in my lunch bag. Some days, when we didn't have food to make lunch, she'd tell me to buy lunch but would still throw a couple cookies in my bag. Ahhhh, how I will miss my wife's daily cookie quota while in Haiti; *do they have cookies in Haiti*, I wonder.

Two weeks without the Southern California sun, dry heat, and family was going to be tough. Albeit home will be dearly missed, I knew going to Haiti was the right thing to do. I wasn't going not because I wanted to, but rather because I *had* to. Something inside me had been kindled after the earthquake. A sense of belonging came to be and I knew I had to go to Haiti to help.

For most people, one trip to Haiti satisfies their need for medical tourism. As it is put, they came, they saw, and they conquered. Not me. After every trip, time blew by as I re-engaged in my busy modern life, but after a few weeks I started feeling the itch. Something inside yearns to return to Haiti, a fire rekindles. I know I will not be satisfied unless I go back. Is it the selfless act of volunteering my time to provide medical care that calls for me? Or is it a selfish need for righting all the wrongs I do while back home? Maybe it is my way of justifying the money I just spent on an Android tablet I know I really do not need, or the watch I bought last weekend at REI. In a way, my trip to Haiti is an amalgam of all of these reasons at the same time, and that is not necessarily a bad thing. In fact, it is what keeps me motivated to go back.

After every trip I've made, I'm happy to come home. Physically tired, dirty, and mentally drained it takes me a few days just to recover. On one trip, a student who accompanied me and stayed for one week summarized her experience as "This whole trip has felt like one long day." I agreed with her. Happy to return to the simple pleasures in life; a warm shower, cutting my toe nails at home, letting my cat drool on my hair, and eating way more calories than I really need meant more every time I returned from that stricken nation.

## What could I do?

I had no prior training in disaster response nor had I ever been to Haiti or the Caribbean. I was not sure how I would be able to handle the situation on the ground. Albeit I did not have much disaster training setting off to Haiti, I was a Family Physician and that would carry me a long way I would soon learn!

As a Family Physician my training is quite global. In my field, I am trained to take care of children and adults (including hospitalized and outpatients), critically ill adults in the intensive care unit, pregnant women and deliveries, and even basic emergency care. Most of us are competent in performing vaginal deliveries and many of us have further training in obstetrics including multiple gestations, high blood pressure or diabetes during pregnancy, and performing cesarean sections. As if that was not enough to know, we are also performing many other procedures such as colonoscopies, circumcisions, basic emergency/trauma care, and other minor surgical procedures. With such a diverse set of skills, we make for an ideal physician for international work as we can truly see any patient that walks in the door and stabilize and manage most medical scenarios.

Within 24 hours after the earthquake, University of Miami/Project Medishare (PM) set up a field-trauma hospital at the request of the Haitian Government on the Port-au-Prince (PaP) airport field where it would stay for months to come. It was with PM that I would travel to Haiti and with my training as a Family Physician that I embarked with the confidence that I had the needed skills to manage whatever walked through the doors.

## Getting Time Off

I had decided that I was to go to Haiti to help in the relief effort but scheduling time to do so would be a feat in and of itself. As a physician, we work some of the longest hours out there. Eighty hours a week is a norm in our field as are 30 hour shifts with no sleep

– sometimes every fourth or fifth night. With that kind of work load, it is quite difficult to schedule time off. Even calling in sick is not simple. When we call in sick, doctors have to be shuffled around from different clinics to ensure there is adequate coverage without compromising patient care. Our patients count on us not getting sick and scheduling leave is not an easy task. Scheduling time off to go to Haiti with such short notice was going to be a challenge.

I would soon be on a hospital rotation block with patients who would be my responsibility. I knew I would have to 'sign out' these patients to another doctor in order to leave for Haiti. 'Sign Out' is a hot issue in medical education and has recently made the news in light of sign out errors. When physicians change shifts they tell the upcoming team of physicians about the patients in the hospital, their plan of treatment, labs/studies which need to be followed up, etc. This is done in a systematic fashion to minimize error between teams, but the system of sign out inherently has risks. Ideally, the sign out would occur between Team A to B and then back from B to A to minimize errors. This, however, is often not the case. Imagine a weekend where there are multiple teams covering the hospital service: Team A signs out to Team B who then signs out to Team C who signs out to Team D who then signs back out to Team B. Each transition point has the potential for error and when done multiple times the risk of error is truly significant. Eventually, the errors add up and patient care may be compromised. Because of past errors leading to injury and even death in some cases, standards have been put in place to prevent and minimize error by ensuring the same few physicians are responsible for patient care. Usually this involves two teams for most inpatient services – a day team and a night team. On the flip side, this two tiered or three tiered approach requires doctors to work more frequent and longer hours – increasing the cycle of fatigue in medicine.

Knowing a bit about the medical system helps the reader to understand how difficult it is to take time off during a patient care cycle. At the time of the earthquake I was on a clinical rotation block which would not allow me to take time off. A bit over a week later, I would start a one month block of obstetrics (OB). OB was a fairly busy block– we worked about 75 hours a week and were on call working 30 hour shifts twice a week. It took a lot of running around and schedule swapping but eventually I was able to take the needed time off. Now that I had the official okay from my boss and time off from work to go, I had to organize myself and purchase needed supplies.

## Gathering Supplies

I had done some reading about supplies needed for relief workers in tropical countries from a few different sources. Based on this information, I pretty much surmised that I was going on a camping trip for some time. We were to sleep on cots in a giant circus tent and our lack of amenities would make Boy Scout summer camp look like a stay at the Ritz Carlton. We may or may not have running water on any given day, food was to be delivered once a day by a local restaurant, and there may be some MRE's (meals ready to eat) donated by the military. I was told there was to be an abundant supply of bottled water at least. I was a boy scout (life scout - one merit badge away from eagle) and camping was nothing new to me. That said, I had not been camping in over 10 years nor had I been camping outside the U.S. This was going to be a whole new experience!

The next few days I worked full time, coming home some days at 8

P.M. Any time away from work was spent gathering a list of supplies. To secure said supplies I went to Big 5, Wal-Mart, and local military surplus stores. My supply list was diverse, including the common list of camping gear and the not so-common such as basic prescriptions to keep myself healthy if I were to get sick in a third world country, malaria prophylaxis, baby wipes, mosquito repellant, iodine tablets to purify water, hundred packets of powdered Gatorade to keep hydrated, boxes of Promax energy bars, and even old floral bed sheets cut up into head bands to stop the sweat from dripping in my eyes. Also on my shopping list were supplies to donate including vitamins (pediatric and prenatal), blankets, clothes, shoes, and medications (prescription and over the counter).

Once the shopping was completed I purchased my plane ticket. I had heard that a few airlines were providing free airfare for medical professionals travelling to Haiti. I contacted United Airlines, American Airlines, and Delta Airlines to ask if they would donate the fare for the trip. As expected from the mega profit greed machine, the airlines all rejected my request. They said they only offered free airfare the first couple of days post-earthquake and now that it was coming on 2 weeks, the airlines no longer thought that volunteers deserved financial assistance in their selfless plight to Haiti – why was I not surprised?

As I was purchasing my supplies and plane ticket to Miami, I contemplated how I was to afford this added expense. Finances for a young physician are tight – school loans, car payment, mortgage, etc. all on a salary just slightly over minimum wage meant we literally lived paycheck to paycheck. I had already spent close to $2000 buying supplies for myself and to donate. I began to seek funds from friends and family and received a tremendous amount of support. In the end, after generous donations I was able to pay my way to Haiti without breaking my bank. Asides from the above supplies, I also was able to secure an overabundance of medications. Friends bought vitamins and medications from Costco and wrote themselves prescriptions so they could donate prescriptions drugs as well as over the counters. One of my friends wrote out almost ten prescriptions for different antibiotics and brought them all in. I wonder what the pharmacist must have thought when she filled all of those meds – enough to pretty much kill every single bacterium she had in her body. Thanks to my colleagues and my father and his colleagues I was able to take over $20,000 worth of medications and donations on my numerous trips.

My father is a veterinarian and growing up as child without health insurance, he was always our primary care provider. If we were sick he would help diagnose us and provide the necessary medications. I remember as a child being given antibiotics by my father which always seemed a bit peculiar. The name sounded familiar: amoxicillin, penicillin, and doxycycline, but the vessel of delivery was quite the opposite. Our pills were always in a red bottle like most others but instead of having the pharmacy name or phone number on the bottle, ours had pictures of dogs, cats, and horses. At first I did not understand the comedy in this but one day I was at school and opened the bottle to take my medications and a friend asked me why I was taking animal pills. Afterschool that day I asked my father why I was taking animal pills and he explained to me that the pills animals take and humans take are the same, just packaged differently and more expensive for the two legged upright ones.

As I gathered supplies for the trip, my father and his colleagues graciously donated hundreds of bottles of medications from their veterinary clinics. For the most part bulk medication bottles (the kinds the pharmacist have in the stock room) are the same between veterinary and human medicine. Bayer makes aspirin for dogs and humans. In fact, the same aspirin your pharmacist would dispense to you, your veterinarian is dispensing for your pet – hence why your dog's last prescription of cipro was so expensive. The medications I had were all in large bulk packaging which would not be amenable to travelling. I would not be able to fit all of these bottles in my luggage. I had to remove the medications and repackage them in zip-lock bags. Luckily my wonderful wife and brother helped and after about four hours, we had all the medications labeled and placed in zip-lock bags ready to pack. This ingenious method of repackaging bulk medications came in handy for multiple trips and saved space in transport.

## Getting There

We were allotted two check-in bags of fifty pounds each for the trip. The night before leaving I pulled two old suitcases I planned to donate. When reading the email, I had mistakenly read that we were allowed 100 pounds per suitcase when in fact it said 100 pounds total. I assumed I would have to pay an overweight baggage fee but didn't want to cut out any of the great donations I had received. I filled one suitcase with my own personal supplies and a few medication bags which came to about 100 pounds. The second suitcase was completely filled with medications alone and was at 100 pounds. On my back was a large Kelty camping backpack which was the only thing I planned to return with.

The flight to Miami was uneventful and went as planned. I came into Miami the night before as the flight to PaP was early in the morning and no flights from the West Coast would make it in time. I stayed the night in a motel, having to lug around over 250 pounds worth of luggage. The next morning I showed up to the Vision airlines desk and checked in with the PM group. When the clerk saw the total weight of my baggage he didn't even ask what was inside. He knew it must have been supplies to donate to Haiti and let the bags go without an added fee. What a surprise!

We were told to arrive at 0600 for a flight that didn't even board until 1200 or so. Those morning hours were thus spent getting to know the other volunteers. I was the only volunteer I had met from the Los Angeles area. Most of the volunteers were from the Miami region. Those of us not from Miami represented the diversity of our country. I had expected most people to be from one of the coasts but in fact the volunteers came from all over the country: Michigan, Oregon, Wisconsin, New York, New Jersey, Texas, and Arizona seemed to be the most represented states. I met physicians, nurses, midwifes, physical/occupational therapists, and support staff all there for the same reason. We had all taken time off, vacation, spent money to get here, and taken a risk in entering a disaster zone with a collapsed infrastructure and sketchy security all for the same reason – to help the Haitians to the best of our ability. It was quite moving and humbling to meet so many selfless people with such great intentions. At that point I knew this was going to be a life changing event for all of us.

Since that first trip there have been many more. I continue to travel to Haiti frequently and take undergraduates, medical students, and physicians in training with me. For most, this is their first experience in a disaster zone and a developing nation. Their reaction is familiar: fear and nervousness transform into confidence and selflessness by the time they leave. As soon as they return they are asking when we can go back. That's Haiti. You go once and you fall in love with the cause, the people, and the country. In this book I will share with you some of the stories that changed our lives - in doing so, I hope it will generate an interest to explore and learn more about our neighbors. Haiti is just one nation suffering - hundreds of others suffer daily with no voice to speak up for them. Please consider donating to organizations working in Haiti, abroad, and in your own country so we can continue to rebuild our world.


Happy reading and God bless us all.

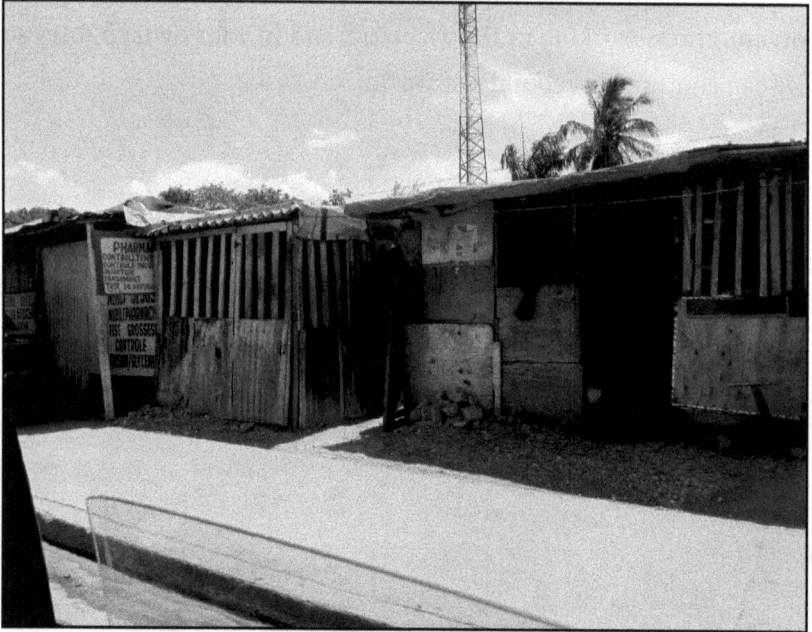
Modified tent city. Two years after the earthquake.

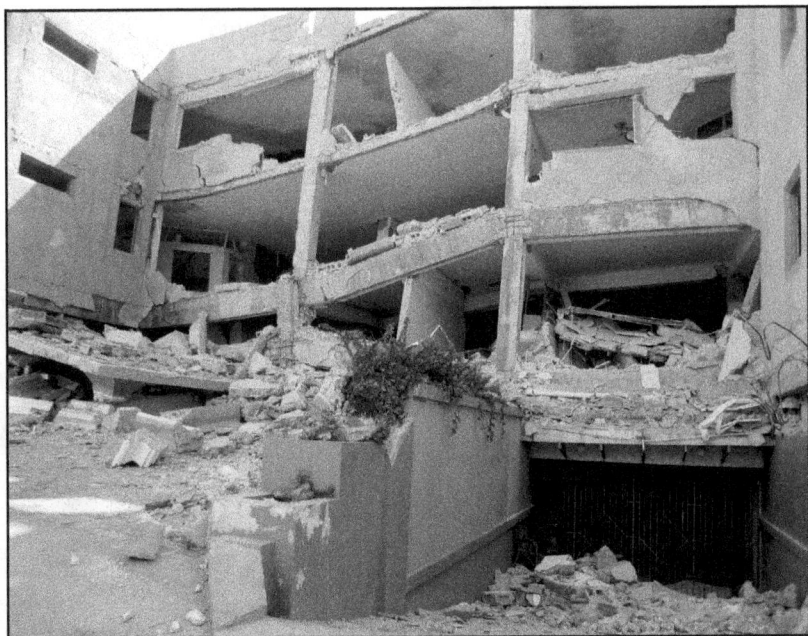

Apartment complex.

# Where's Haiti?

*Life is an opportunity, benefit from it.*
*Life is beauty, admire it.*
*Life is a dream, realize it.*
*Life is a challenge, meet it.*
*Life is a duty, complete it.*
*Life is a game, play it.*
*Life is a promise, fulfill it.*
*Life is sorrow, overcome it.*
*Life is a song, sing it.*
*Life is a struggle, accept it.*
*Life is a tragedy, confront it.*
*Life is an adventure, dare it.*
*Life is luck, make it.*
*Life is too precious, do not destroy it.*
*Life is life, fight for it.*

- Mother Teresa -

# The Earthquake

What were you doing on Tuesday, the 12th of January, 2010 at 21:53:10 UTC (approximately 5 PM EST)? Were you at work? Were you at the gym? Shopping? Lunch? Checking your stocks? Most of us can't pinpoint a specific memory to that time as we were busy in our everyday dealings. For millions of Haitians, however, they can't forget when a 7.2 magnitude earthquake changed their world.

I was in clinic seeing a patient when my cell phone started vibrating. Actively engaged in patient care, I ignored the alert. I suspected it was a text from my wife asking about dinner or what she should wear to work. A few minutes later I stepped aside into my work area and pulled my phone out of its belt holster and the alert I read took me by surprise. It was a breaking news alert from BBC News and it read "Breaking News: Magnitude 7.2 Earthquake Devastates Port-Au-Prince, Haiti." I shuddered upon reading the notification – having been raised and living in Southern California, earthquakes are nothing new to me, but a magnitude 7.2 puts even a Californian on edge (later confirmed by United States Geological Society, USGS, as a 7.0).

A few months prior I was working on the Sixth floor of Harbor-UCLA Medical Center in the South Bay of Southern California when the Northern Baja California quake of magnitude 5.9 hit on the 30th of December, 2009. I was sitting on an office chair with wheels writing a progress note in a chart, updating the events of the day for the medical records. Working long hours as a physician often tests our senses. Sometimes even walking after a 30 hour shift is a daunting task and the simple activity of lifting one's foot and putting it back down becomes a major feat. It can be likened to the feeling of walking on dry land after being on a boat for a few hours.

As I was writing my progress note in the morning, I felt a bit off balance. It seemed like the room was spinning - I could not figure out what was the matter. I wondered if I had too much coffee. As I sat there contemplating why I felt dizzy, I began to realize that the whole chair was swaying to and fro on its wheels. At that point I realized I was riding an earthquake. Riding an earthquake wave in a seismic retrofitted building is quite exciting to say the least – the entire building swayed back and forth on its rollers and I just sat there and enjoyed the ride. The quake itself only lasted about 15 or 20 seconds but thanks to the building's seismic rollers, the ride kept going for about a minute or so. Once the shaking subsided, I looked outside – everything seemed ok. I went to the USGS website (a favorite bookmarked site for many Californians) and looked up the data: 5.9 magnitude with an epicenter in the Baja region of Northern Mexico.

I tried calling my family to make sure everyone was okay but could not get through. I assumed cellular phone companies block non-essential calls during emergencies to keep the system from getting overloaded and hindering availability to emergency access numbers. After a couple of minutes of trying, I presumed the above and resorted to texting loved ones which seems to work fine during times like this. A few minutes later I was able to confirm that everyone was doing fine and we all moved on with our day, prepared for a few aftershocks here and there but nothing to slow our daily progress.

That was a 5.9 magnitude earthquake which gave us all a pretty fun roller coaster ride, and left cracks in a few buildings. So shouldn't a 7.0 be just a tad worse? It is only 1.1 points higher right? Truth be told, a 1.1 difference is actually quite significant and makes a 7.0 magnitude over 12 times stronger than a 5.9 magnitude quake. One would need 44 5.9 magnitude earthquakes to equal the power quite released from a 7.0 magnitude earthquake. Why such a difference? Well, the answer lay within the mathematics of how the moment magnitude scale (MMS) works. There are other ways of measuring earthquake intensity including the Richter scale but for the most part the MMS is the common modality of measurement, having overtaken the Richter scale a few years ago. The MMS is a base-10 to the 1.5 logarithmic scale, meaning every increase in 1 on the scale corresponds to an increase in $10^{1.5}$ times of the respective item. Thus, a difference in magnitude of 1.1 corresponds to about 44 times more energy released from the quake as compared to the 5.9 – wow!

The last large earthquake many of us can recall in the United States was the magnitude 6.9 Loma Prieta earthquake of California in 1989. The earthquake struck at 17:04 PM PST during the baseball world series in the Bay Area, lasted 10-15 seconds, and devastated Northern California. Fifty-seven people died directly from the earthquake and another six from subsequent related conditions or injuries and anywhere from 6,000 to 12,000 people were left homeless. Luckily the traffic conditions were lighter than usual due to the World Series of Baseball (San Francisco Giants VS Oakland Athletics). Given the local rivalries, many people stayed home or at viewing parties for the game. This quake was strong enough to collapse the Bay Bridge leading to one fatality. The iconic images of cars sandwiched by concrete on the bridge are engrained in our memories. If the traffic had been as heavy as usual for a Tuesday evening (rush hour), many more likely would have perished. The damage totaled $6 billion – making it one of the most expensive natural disasters in U.S. history at that time, and led to numerous new retrofitting and building codes.

Looking down at my phone and reading the news alert in light of the memories of the 6.9 Loma Prieta quake and riding the 5.9 quake in the hospital, I shuddered. I could not begin to fathom the level of destruction a developing nation would endure with such a strong quake. As soon as things settled down in the hospital I checked National Public Radio's website and saw the details: 7.0, Port-Au Prince, Haiti, buildings completely demolished, power outage across the city, fires, wounded in the streets. The magnitude 7.0 earthquake struck at 21:53 UTC (16:53 local time) about 16 miles west of Port-au-Prince. The earthquake itself lasted 10-15 seconds but the shaking continued for about 30-40 seconds.

I later learned from local Haitian construction workers that authorities seldom enforced building code and standards, thus the minimum building standard wasn't really a minimum nor was it a standard. To save money, many people used unsafe practices of diluting concrete mix. One worker told me he mixed concrete with sand to save money. One bag of concrete would last three times as long but the resultant structure was much more brittle. Normally, to prevent concrete shearing, pieces of steel are placed in the concrete called rebar (reinforcement bar). Most building codes require or recommend notched rebar instead of smooth rebar as it provides more support within concrete. In Haiti, notched rebar was about twice the cost of smooth rebar due to the additional step needed in its manufacturing. Many buildings were thus built with brittle concrete and smooth rebar, making the buildings apt to crumble when stressed – hence why buildings literally crumbled during the earthquake.

The USGS recorded over eight major aftershocks in the two hours post-quake. These shocks were anywhere between 4.3 and 5.9. Each aftershock was the magnitude of the Loma Prieta quake itself. Those who had survived the main earthquake had not anticipated the strong aftershocks and many perished when further buildings collapsed that people were seeking refuge in. When the shaking subsided, the resultant devastation left would scar the country and bring Haiti into the international spotlight.

---

"Where's Haiti?", one of my classmates once asked me years before the earthquake during a book review/discussion of Tracy Kidder's *Mountains Beyond Mountains* in medical school. My answer was as blunt and honest as I could be "I don't know where the heck Haiti is, I think it's somewhere in the Caribbean." Before we could go on and 'Wiki' or 'Google' it, the moderator jumped in and redirected our conversation. We then continued our discussion of Dr. Paul Farmer's expeditions to Haiti. For those who are unaware of Dr. Farmer's medical service in Haiti, *Mountains Beyond Mountains* is an excellent synopsis of his personal quest and the humanitarian efforts of the organization Partners in Health (PIH). PIH does tremendous work in Haiti, medically and socially, and have made huge leaps and bounds in the treatment of MDR TB (multidrug resistant Tuberculosis).

After our discussion and reading of *Mountains Beyond Mountains* I knew a bit about the TB problem plaguing Haiti but that was about it. We were all busy keeping our heads above water in medical school and Haiti got tucked away in the back of my mind. Years later as I read the BBC text alert on my phone describing the earthquake that never answered question resurfaced at the tip of my tongue: *Where's Haiti and how can I help*, I said aloud.

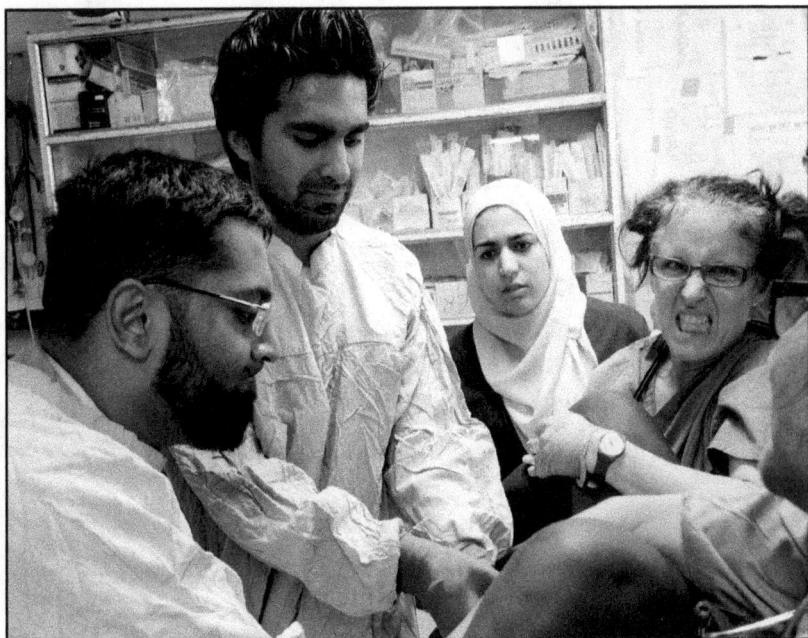
Team effort in delivering a healthy baby.

# The Aftermath

*There are only two ways to live your life. One is as though nothing is a miracle. The other is as though everything is a miracle.*

- Albert Einstein -

For millions of people an event which lasted seconds changed their lives forever. Millions displaced, hundreds of thousands dead, rubble everywhere. Can you imagine such a catastrophe occurring in your home country? How would your society deal with no running water or food for days? These were the thoughts running through my mind as I pondered what the Haitians must be experiencing.

Hours after the quake, news came from PaP detailing the fires, deaths and people trapped in buildings. The infrastructure of Haiti was weak to begin with and had now completely collapsed. Hospitals in and around the city were destroyed or significantly damaged. The airport was scarred as was the seaport, thus limiting the ability of aid to enter the country by traditional means of transport. Roads were blocked with debris and bodies. People were buried under rubble. It was hell.

The trademark picture of damage from the earthquake broadcasted by the major news networks was that of The National Palace. The National Palace sustained significant damage with large portions of the complex having collapsed to the ground (the presidential family was safe). The PaP prison sustained enough damage to allow 4000 inmates to escape. It was estimated that 250,000 residences and 30,000 commercial buildings were damaged significantly and required demolition. In less than one minute, over one million people were made homeless and the quake led to 230,000 deaths and about 300,000 injuries. To better comprehend this number, imagine all the homes in Detroit, Michigan suddenly vanishing (population 951,270) and leaving the entire populace of Detroit homeless. This was the situation Haiti was now faced with.

Families abroad had no way of knowing if their loved ones were safe. The public telephone system was down so there was no means of open communication. All communication was forwarded via the emergency broadcast stations but the general radio stations were off air for over a week. Cellular phone service was disrupted. Digicel and Comcel (two of PaP's major cellular providers) reported outages due to damage to their cellular towers. It took days for the cellular system to be operational and weeks for the rest of the communication facilities to come back on air.

President René Préval declared a national emergency and made an appeal for humanitarian aid. The first country to provide aid was neighboring Dominican Republic (D.R.). The D.R. sent much needed water, food, machinery for lifting and transporting rubble, and medical supplies. They organized medical teams and opened up their own hospitals for transporting patients to the D.R. who needed advanced medical care.

Parliament was shattered, many of its members dead or injured. As a result of the lack of communication, the president was not able to fully determine who was heading the rescue mission. There were daily meetings between the president and the United Nations (UN) to coordinate activities for the day. However, with communication down, roadways blocked, and members of government missing, the resultant chaos led to looting and violence. Stores where people went to stock up on precious supplies such as water, toilet paper, food, and medication were looted first. Electronic stores and shopping centers were also looted. Violent acts occurred. People were desperate, and in times of desperation people often resort to tactics they would not consider otherwise.

People had nowhere to go and no one to call for help. Even if they were able to call, there was no way for help to get to them those first few critical hours. While foreign and domestic assistance was being organized, people tried pulling their loved ones from the rubble. They were forced to sleep in the streets with only the clothes they had on their backs. Ordinary citizens became heroes as they helped each other out of the rubble and out of harm's way. The first responders were not professional search and rescue teams, but were in fact Haitian residents who came to each other's aid that first day.

The Dominican Red Cross partnered with the International Red Cross in sending aid urgently. Within the first few weeks of the quake the D.R. had sent hundreds of trucks across its borders carrying food, medicine, medical personnel, and humanitarian supplies. They helped establish some of the first feeding stations and clean water stations. It is estimated that their cooks were cooking over 100,000 meals a day from their mobile kitchens.

The second day post-earthquake, urban search and rescue teams from the U.S., Cuba, and other nearby countries including the D.R. arrived. These teams came equipped with heavy machinery, search dogs, audio search technology, and other needed supplies. However, with debris scattered across the road, use of heavy machinery initially proved more difficult than anticipated. Therefore, much of the initial rescue effort was done by hand. One medical provider who was an ex-army trauma physician told me his story:

*I was already in PaP working on medical relief when the earthquake hit. I remember being in the lunch hall of our building at the time of the event and running outside for safety. It sounded like a freight train was driving through our complex. The Earth was rolling beneath me and I just squatted down and rode the wave, kinda like surfing. All around me I could see people running, screaming and confused.*

*Once the earthquake was done, I looked back and the lunch hall had collapsed and I was covered in dust. I was in shock and just walked around for the first couple of minutes. The dormitories were still intact and after a few minutes of taking in the scene, I went to my room and pulled out my medical bag which had supplies like tourniquets and scalpels, morphine, and a few other medications.*

*I began administering basic field first aid and triaging. Lots of people had broken bones, bleeding wounds, and many were trapped in the rubble. It seemed like only 5 minutes but hours had gone by and finally I went to the neighboring homes to help out as well. I didn't sleep that night; I just kept working to keep people alive.*

*The next day I heard an announcement on the radio that emergency response units were only now being mobilized and parts of the city were isolated due to damaged roads and fires.*

*There were many people trapped under debris. We started intravenous fluids, gave them plenty of pain medications and tried to manually clear the debris. If I didn't get them out soon they would die* from kidney failure or shock. After a few hours we finally gave up on removing them and I knew they didn't have long to live if they stayed pinned under the rubble.

I had a shitty decision to make – there were people trapped in the rubble with severe crush injuries and we couldn't manually extract them. I didn't know if and when professional rescue squads would make it to this side of town. Either I went out there and amputated limbs to extract them or they would die. I decided the uncertainty of waiting was too great and had to get them out of there. I'll never forget what I had to do next. In all my years of military trauma including field deployments in Iraq and Afghanistan I had never seen trauma to this extent. I literally gave people 15 or 20 milligrams of Morphine to ease some pain [most people require 2-4mg of morphine to reduce pain] and took out my trauma kit and did amputations with a hemostat, scalpel, portable cautery, and trauma saw.

It was the most grotesque situation I had ever been in but our actions saved their lives since it took 2 weeks for heavy machinery to make it to our part of town.

Many of those I saved are now my best friends, amputees yes, but alive – and we're all grateful for that.

---

We have all smelled burning hair at some point – it has quite a distinct pungent smell that etches itself into our memories. Now imagine that smell exponentially multiplied – how would that smell to you? Morgues were overflowing with bodies and were not equipped to handle a disaster of this scale. People began stacking body parts and bodies on the streets and public areas. About two weeks post-quake, the government had organized trucks to pick up the bodies and place them in mass graves. As they began to run out of room, many bodies were simply burned in the streets. By this time, the bodies had already spent a significant amount of time out in the Caribbean sun and humidity, bringing a putrid smell to the region. Haiti was literally rotting.

Hospitals that survived the quake were quickly over burdened with patients. Every inch of these hospitals were occupied, including patients sleeping in the restrooms with intravenous fluid bags hanging. One physician I had worked with told me he was doing amputations in the kitchen area of a small hospital as there was no room elsewhere. He used a cooking pot to catch the amputated body part and blood.

Four days after the quake, on January 16th, President Préval handed over control of the PaP airport to the U.S. The Haitians were unable to manage air traffic in and out of the air space since their air traffic control tower was leveled during the quake. Five days post-earthquake medical supplies began to run low. Antibiotics, pain medications, intravenous fluids and other supplies which were able to be salvaged from amongst the rubble began to dwindle. The Director of Partners in Health (Ophelia Dahl) said "…as many as 20,000 people will die each day that could have been saved by surgery." Medical providers were left with little supplies to treat patients with. The fifth day was also about the time when major helicopter aid drops and aid ships/

supplies began to arrive in PaP.

Day 11, January 23rd, the Haitian government officially called off the search and rescue phase and began the recovery phase for bodies. By this point the probability of finding survivors was miniscule. Many countries had provided medical teams and supplies which were now being organized and distributed by various organizations. Project Medishare had established a tent hospital on the grounds of the PaP airport with 300 beds, an intensive care unit, emergency department, physical and rehabilitation services, a pediatric ward, a trauma bay, and an operating room. This was one of the most well equipped hospitals and the *first* trauma and rehabilitation hospital in Haiti. By February, less than four weeks after the earthquake, Project Medishare had a fully functioning hospital being run out of tents. It was with Project Medishare that I would find my way to Haiti.

In a matter of seconds an already impoverished Haiti was devastated. A proud society was left begging for assistance from the international community. Aid did indeed come but not fast enough for many. In those first eleven days close to 300,000 people died and over two million were left homeless and displaced on the streets of PaP. In only seconds what took generations to build was wiped out. Recovery would be a long and arduous process.

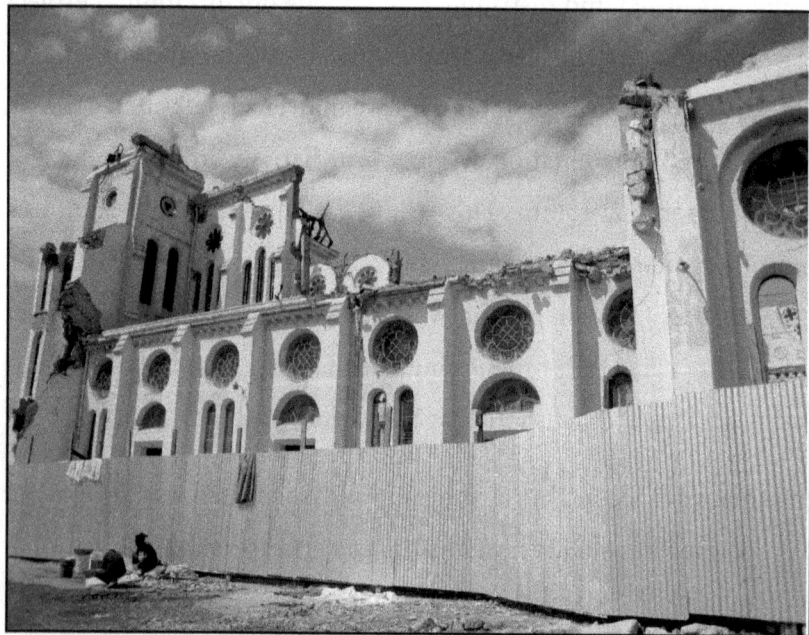

Cathedral of Our Lady of the Assumption. Built between 1884 and 1914, this cathedral stood as a beacon to mariners entering the port. Destroyed during the quake, the Archbishop and others died inside.

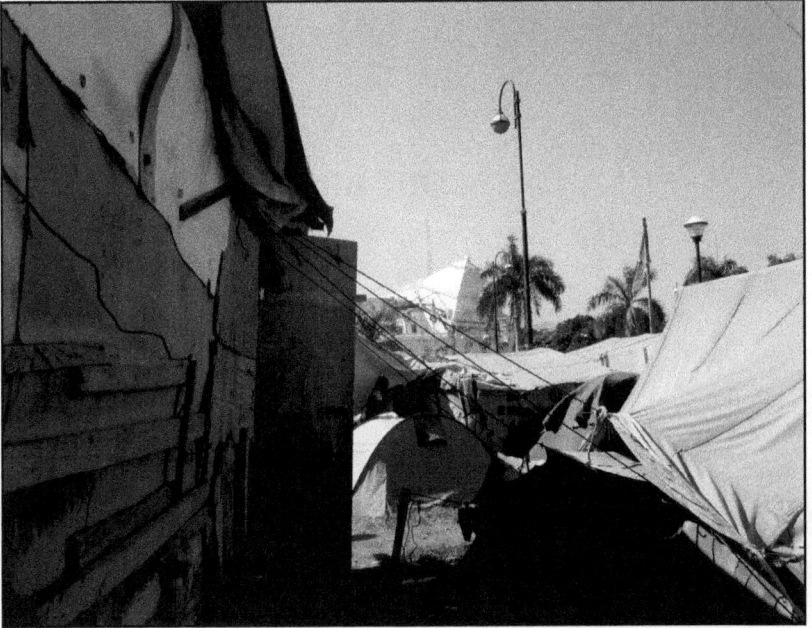

Tent city at the city center. Note the proximity of the collapsed capital building in the background.

# Bienvenue à Haïti!

*Adversity is the diamond dust Heaven polishes its jewels with.*

- Thomas Carlyle -

Ready to help, I had my bags packed with donated and purchased medications and supplies. I carried with me the end result and intent of hundreds of people who had donated money and supplies to help the Haitians. Even though I was only one person, I brought with me the energy of hundreds. Knowing so many had selflessly given so much helped motivate me as I readied to leave. I walked out of my front door in Southern California with two large suitcases and a backpack ready for anything and everything.

The hardest part of that first trip was the day I left home. For five years of marriage, other than being on call, I had never spent more than a couple nights away from my wife. Even when I had been on call or my wife went to visit her family in Northern California I knew we were close. If there was an emergency I was just a few hours' drive or an hour flight away at most. Now, however, I was heading out to a new frontier – a seven hour flight and far enough that I lost that omnipresent sense of security for the first time. Yet something pulled me out that door and on my journey. My wife, parents, and brother all provided a new sense of support with their well wishes, thoughts, and prayers. Anxious, scared, and excited I boarded my planed and was off to Miami, and from there, PaP.

## Touchdown

During the flight from Miami to PaP I continued to wonder what I would see. I was not sure what to expect and hoped that I had brought everything needed. Was I going to be able to make a difference? How would this trip change me? These are but a few of the questions which raced through my mind. The flight from

Miami to PaP was actually quite pleasant and short. From takeoff to touchdown we were in flight for less than two hours. As we were flying in, I looked out the window and could see the coast and the port. Numerous naval ships were docked at the port. From this distance the ships were surreal, like children's toys floating in a bathtub. Nothing seemed real or tangible quite yet from 15,000 feet in the air.

As the land began to come into view, I could see the brown color of the Earth and scattered patches of white and green slowly appearing. Approaching the landing strip, what initially appeared to be vague white patches became more discernible as housing. Once we were on our final approach the houses were clear enough to make out some detail. I was able to see homes and the roads leading to them along with the clothes lines hanging on top. The most detail I could make out were the large black and red water reservoirs that sat atop these buildings. At this distance, everything seemed to be at peace – the antithesis of what I had seen on television. I then started to notice that about half of the white patches were really more brownish-white and uneven in shape. As the homes came in closer view the picture became clear – even from the sky the damage was obvious. The brown that I was seeing was in fact rubble and crumbled homes and buildings. Almost half of the homes I could see were destroyed. Others had noticed the devastation as well and an encompassing noise was heard throughout the plane as hundreds of us gasped at what lay beneath. It was Haiti's emergency flare – the land was calling me, inviting me, welcoming me in to help. I felt the first rush of adrenaline as the situation finally hit me. Chills ran down my spine and I knew I was supposed to be here.

As we were landing I pondered what I would see. How does one prepare for entering a third world disaster zone for the first time? As the plane touched down, what I saw surprised me: the landscape was surreally familiar. It looked just like the landscape back home. The shrubs and small trees that lined the water rich semi-arid regions of Texas or California came to mind. I had expected a starkly different land, maybe something out of a "Save Ethiopia" fundraising telethon with a barren landscape and scattered mud huts. Surprisingly Haiti looked much like what I was familiar to. Travelling has always been a passion of mine and in every country visited, I had expected the people and the land to be very different – almost alien like. Yet as I saw Haiti for the first time I realized that in all my travels I had not been able to pinpoint any major differences between cultures and places. We are all human and this is one Earth after all. The similarities vastly outnumbered the differences. I had not even disembarked the plane yet and Haiti had already taught me my first lesson: she was not that different than home.

The landing strip was relatively unscathed and while taxiing, the rest of the airport came into view. The site of green military tents and armored U.S. military vehicles were abundant. Planes were unloading cargo marked "USAID." A few other planes including United and Delta airlines were transporting aid workers and U.S. Haitians. Shattered glass and debris lay all over the ground. Foreign soldiers were busy unloading goods from the military helicopters across the field. I assumed these helicopters must be transporting material from the aircraft carriers in the port. A mobile staircase came to the jet door to greet us as our plane came to a stop. We all gathered our belongings and readied to depart the plane. Upon reaching the door, the humidity and smell that are typical of a tropical region hit me full force. It was about ten in the morning, I took a deep breath in and I could already feel myself starting to sweat. My glasses half fogged up as soon as I stepped on the causeway. I had arrived in Haiti at last and found that it was not that different than home and other places I had travelled – quite a reassuring welcome indeed; I was just hoping for a tad less humidity.

## Customs

My first few steps in Haiti were on an old and chipped runway, a sign of the rugged road that lay ahead. The runway seemed to have made it through the earthquake; however the airport was not as lucky. The airport building was in one piece but the large glass viewpoints were shattered. Inside, debris scattered the hallways. My welcome to Haiti began with crumbled buildings and would continue to be scattered with roadblocks and struggles.

To the North of the airport were rolling foothills, brown and lush. The hills were about 2000 feet of elevation. The hilly landscape and humidity was romantic in a sense – simple and beautiful. I imagined in my mind the lush tobacco and sugar cane fields that the locals harvested plentifully decades ago. Following the rolling hills westward the military tents and tarps came into view with the standard olive drab and desert brown designs. There were U.S. military personnel, transport vehicles, helicopters, and US Military C-5 Galaxy transport

*Bienvenue à Haïti!*

aircraft parked in the vicinity. The Galaxy is what its name implies, that is, it is a massive plane made by Lockheed. If you've ever had the opportunity to see one in person it is an awe inspiring site. The plane is about three-quarters the length of a football field and pondering how this behemoth gets off the ground and defies gravity is amazing. From the gut of this beast, foreign workers were actively unloading USAID boxes – the hull almost completely full of them.

I was directed to a large hangar about 200 yards away. Walking to the hangar, I took in my surroundings. There were boxes and boxes of aid needing to be unloaded but there did not seem to be any sense of rush or urgency amongst the local workers. It was a stark difference from what I had just seen in the hull of the C-5. There were some Haitians sitting on the cargo palates playing cards, another group sharing what appeared to be coffee from a thermos, and one person operating a forklift actively unloading the palates with no spotter. It seemed that the acuity of the earthquake had settled in and people were now just going about their normal lives. Just like workers in any country, without adequate supervision and management the labor seemed to move uncoordinated and slow.

Upon reaching the hangar we were directed to walk inside to the makeshift Haitian Customs Desk. There was a large desk with one worker handing out visa forms for us to fill out. Once we obtained our forms, we then walked to an area where four small desks were set up with boxes on either side to regulate the flow of traffic. We were instructed by our group leader on how to fill out the visa forms. Given it was only a couple weeks after the earthquake, the Customs officers wasted no time letting us through. We brought our visas to the officers who gave our passports and paperwork a cursory glance, provided the necessary stamp, and returned the papers to us saying "Merci, Bienvenue à Haïti!" So far so good, I thought.

## Getting to Base Camp

I thought there would be a carousel bringing over my luggage but there were no carousels in this hangar/makeshift airport. There was a door on the far side of the hangar from which workers were unloading baggage by hand off a truck. They placed the baggage inside the hangar and it was a free for all trying to find which bag belonged to whom. I grabbed my bags and put them aside. As I began sifting through the rapidly growing mound of luggage, our group leader made an announcement that our bags would be brought to camp directly in a few hours and we were to exit the hangar and proceed to the front gate. We left our baggage in an area where one of the hospital staff members was collecting them and worked our way outside.

In the hangar, external sounds and smells were relatively minimal and we had no idea what was happening just outside. As we walked to the exit of the hangar the ambient noise and smell from outside began to trickle in. Slowly, the noise and smell grew to something I was quite familiar with – it was an environment I had experienced numerous times before. It smelled like India and Mexico – it smelled like any other developing nation did. There was a must to the odor that can be likened to sweaty gym clothes dipped in kerosene and diesel that began to permeate my senses. The noises became discernible:

48                                           *Bienvenue à Haïti!*

the high pitch and overused horn, traffic, moving vehicles, buzzing from the bicycle wheels, screeching from mopeds, and an amalgam of the voices of hundreds of people peddling goods, offering rides, and arguing. In a way, the familiarity of the symphony that is a metropolitan city in a developing nation was quite calming – I was familiar with this environment and was comforted in identifying the similarities.

Just outside the hangar was a gated area where we were told to wait for our vans to take us to base camp. As we waited, other passengers exited the gate and left the airport. A few feet in front of us was the main road where people had their cars and taxis parked. Peddlers had small trinkets they were selling and others were selling some type of meat product and other snacks and drinks. Everybody had shirts on that said Nike, Reebok, Ralph Lauren, or another brand name of some sort. The logos and text all had some hint of their not so official origin with some being slightly off center and some even being misspelled (Tommy *Hillfiger* instead of *Hilfiger*). Surprisingly though, I did not see many beggars asking for money – possibly due to the plentitude of armed personnel patrolling the airport entrance/ exit, providing international travelers with a false sense of security. Not only were Haitian police in the vicinity, but the UN had a strong presence guarding the gate. Was I to take this as a good sign of stability or a bad omen of the need for all this security? I would find out soon enough.

One small van and two SUVs with the PM logo on their hoods came by every ten minutes or so to pick up a group of us. Our base camp must not be far since the drivers were coming back fairly quickly. After waiting about 35 minutes, it was my turn. We were herded into a vehicle equivalent in size to the old Mazda MPVs from the 90's. Eleven of us were packed tight into a vehicle designed to seat seven. In the third row sat three of us. We sat tight and the two of us on either end were pretty much sitting sideways with one hip on the chair and the other hip facing the ceiling. In the middle row was a similar seating arrangement but a larger seat with five people crammed in. The passenger seat had two people sharing the space. In the end, the driver was the lucky one having his own seat. We were packed in tighter then a can of sardines; if there were an accident, we were not going anywhere. The driver kindly kept the windows rolled down as to prevent suffocation on our own body odor. Once the doors closed, we were off.

The van turned around and we drove by stands with people selling food, small paintings, jewelry, and clothes. The buildings on this street were all relatively intact and were one story shacks and offices. Trash littered the sides of the road and scrawny street dogs were digging through the piles of litter for something to eat. Between food stands were burning piles of rubbish. The smell was suffocating yet alluring at the same time: the raw smell of burning rubber and trash with a hint of the neighbor's grilled chicken. The airport had a brick wall about eight feet tall surrounding the perimeter which had seen its fair share of graffiti. We traveled about half a mile and pulled into a gated entrance back on to the airport, guarded by three armed guards who carried what appeared to be 30 year old sawed off shotguns. Over the brick fence and through the steel gate I could see what looked like three giant circus tents. The driver drove past the second gate which was not guarded and into the complex. We passed a large mango tree and continued around to the front of the tents. There we disembarked our vehicle and joined with the rest of the group on the PM campus – the adventure had officially begun.

## The Tent

When we arrived at the camp, we were instructed to pick a cot in the main sleeping tent. I walked in and was blown away by the sight. I had never seen anything like it before. It felt as if I had entered a circus tent. Were there elephants on the other side and did I bring peanuts? The inside length of the tent was about that of a standard basketball court and was about 80 feet in length. There were six rows of cots lined up right next to each other totaling close to 100 sleeping spaces. Looking down I saw the natural dirt ground and looking up could see some holes in the tent top. The scenario reminded me of something I expected to see on a military boot camp recruit show on the Discovery channel.

These tents were donated by the U.S. FEMA (Federal Emergency Management Agency). Towards the entrance at the front of the tent was an area with sleeping bags, clothes, mosquito nets, twine, soap, shampoo, and other hygienic supplies. Adjacent to this area was a cot with boxes on it filled with MRE's (meals ready to eat) and snacks donated by the U.S. military. Towards the middle-front of the tent were a microwave, coffee maker, and laptop. There were two power bars on the ground with cell phones and a camera battery charging. Ironically, even in such basic living conditions we could not part from our technology. No matter we were in a disaster stricken country with a crumbled infrastructure - we needed our coffee, Facebook, and smartphone!

We were told that we had some time before our official welcome and to relax or explore the campus. It was lunch time and a local Haitian restaurant supplied lunch in a white Styrofoam box. Turns out every day during lunch the restaurant would bring some form of mystery meat, beans, and rice. Some brave souls ate the food and others declined and ate MRE's or snack bars.

As a Muslim, we are encouraged to eat halal meat and thus this practically makes me a vegetarian when I am out. Meat is deemed halal by the way it is killed, similar to kosher meat. The animal is slaughtered while God's name and a small prayer of thanks is said. Back home, food products such as tortillas and beans often use animal based ingredients without explicitly mentioning this. For example, many tortillas and beans use lard and I have ordered numerous "vegetarian salads" which conveniently had bacon on the salad. Most people don't immediately identify animal based ingredients or bacon as "meat." From extensive experience being cautions with what I ate, I knew that no matter what the server says, there is always a chance of meat or meat products being in the food. The clear exception is a restaurant that explicitly markets itself as a vegetarian or vegan. In cases where no halal food is available, it is acceptable to eat kosher or non-halal meat. However, it is still NOT acceptable to consume pork or pork products. Looking at the Styrofoam box my stomach began speaking to me. It reminded me that I had not eaten since the night before and now it was 12:30 in the afternoon. In the box was a meat which looked like either chicken or pork (or maybe an amalgam of the two), beans, and white rice. I knew the Haitian diet was rich in pork so did not want to test the meat and the beans most likely were cooked with lard or a meat sauce. Prepared for this, I grabbed a Promax energy bar from my bag, gave my meal away to a local worker, and began to explore the campus.

## Hospital Bernard Mevs

The tent field hospital was a disaster response hospital providing acute care. As the situation stabilized, there needed to be a more permanent and lasting center. University of Miami/Project Medishare partnered with The Bernard Mevs Group to purchase, renovate, and open the Hospital Bernard Mevs/Project Medishare (HBMPM). The buildings on campus of HBMPM are rather old, having been a prior hospital in the past. An ER, inpatient ward, ICU, pediatrics building, radiology/lab suite, spinal cord unit, isolation rooms, well equipped operating rooms, and outpatient clinics were all organized and located on campus.

Relative to the tent-field hospital, the difference between that and HBMPM was night and day. We had more labs, imaging, an equipped ER, operating rooms, an ICU with ventilators, and even a newly donated CT scanner. HBMPM was now one of the best equipped public trauma and critical care hospitals in all of PaP. The philosophy of HBMPM was that of sustainability. Volunteers coming from the U.S. not only cared for patients but worked closely with the local Haitian nurses, physicians, and staff. Together, the team taught each other new skills, leading to an exchange of knowledge that went well beyond the treatment of any one or two patients a provider could do on their own. Together, we stood in the trenches shoulder to shoulder with our Haitian colleagues in the battle for Haiti.

And with that, I began seeing patients.

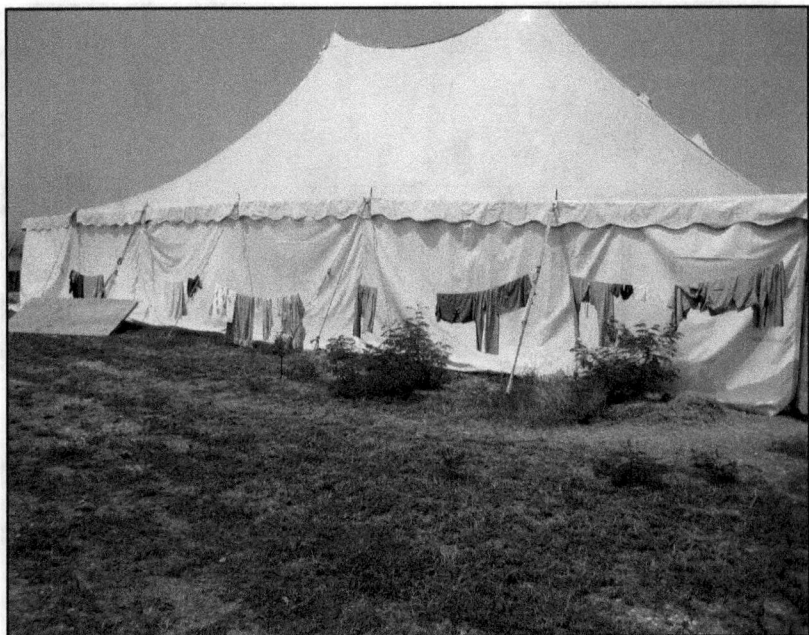

Large FEMA 'circus tent'. One tent was for volunteers to sleep and there were two that functioned as the hospital.

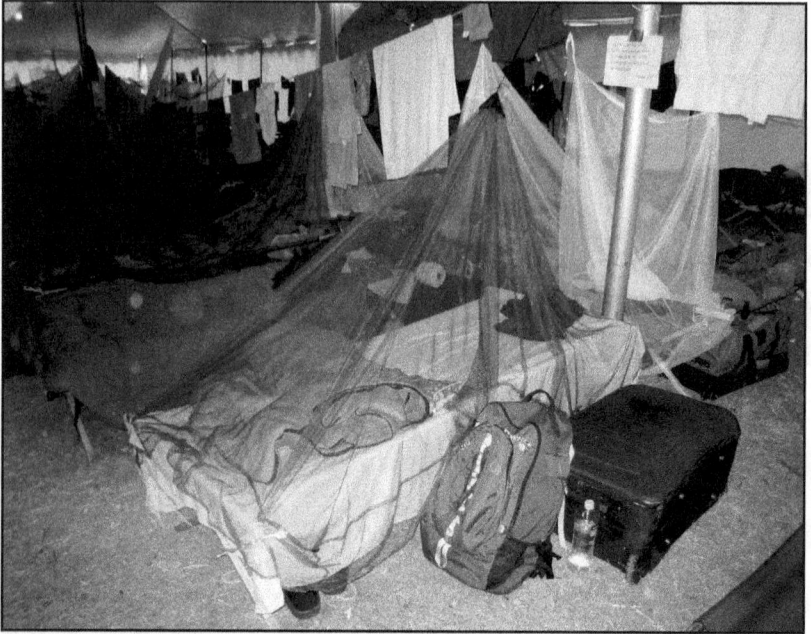

Volunteer sleeping tent.

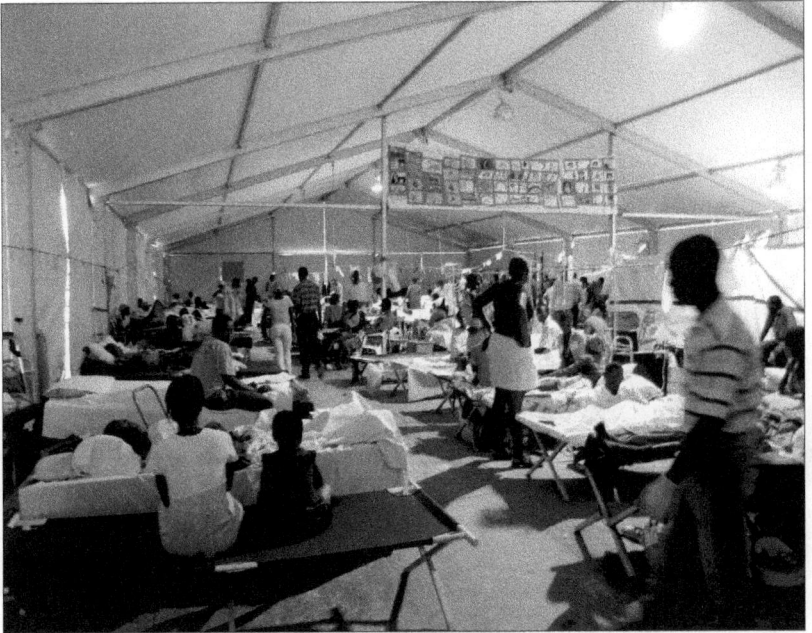

Medical ward tent.

# The Loa

*Christian, Jew, Muslim, shaman, Zoroastrian, stone, ground,*
*mountain, river, each has a secret way of being with the mystery,*
*unique and not to be judged.*


- Rumi -

# Epilepsy

We have known of epilepsy, a type of seizure disorder, for thousands of years. The word itself comes from the Greek *epilambánein*, meaning "to take hold of." When the term was coined, ancient Greek physicians believed the soul was under attack by demons and demigods. As a matter of fact, Hippocrates—yes, the same old doctor for which the Hippocratic oath is dubbed, the oath all doctors still take—called epilepsy the "sacred disease," implying a battle between good and evil within the body.

The Greeks weren't the only ones to attribute seizures to the supernatural. Throughout history, many cultures blamed spirits and demons. The ancient Babylonians, Romans, Egyptians, Chinese, and Indus civilizations pinned the cause on deities. As modern medicine evolved, so did our understanding of this disease. To this day, many cultures believe that seizures are a result of spirit or demonic possession. Anne Fadiman authored the best seller *The Spirit Catches You and You Fall Down*, a true story which accounts the life of Lia Lee, a Hmong child born with a seizure disorder. The family truly believes that the child is being contacted by spirits, and through time, those touched by spirits gain an understanding of the ephemeral world and eventually become shamans. Thus they are hesitant at obtaining western allopathic treatment until forced to as this isn't necessarily a bad thing in their view. Through cultural miscommunication, use of inappropriate homeopathic and allopathic cures, and recurrent seizures, young Lia's brain is starved of oxygen from these attacks and she finally becomes cognitively impaired and has permanent brain damage. This excellent story details the cultural complexity in treating a patient whose culture understands a problem in a different way than Western thought. In this case, unfortunately for Lia, the outcome was not what anyone had hoped for.

Through decades of research and ill-fated treatments for seizures, such as drilling holes in patients' heads to let out the bad spirits, we now understand that epilepsy is a disease in which a region of the brain does not follow the rules. The brain is basically a large computer. Like a computer, the brain is an array of circuitry. Cells act like circuits. Nerves are the wires connecting the circuits to one another. Like computers, brain cells talk to each other via electrical signals. The electrical impulses are sent in an organized fashion, with certain regions of the brain responsible for certain activities and thoughts. This organized activity allows the brain to perform complex computational tasks—input information, analyze it and output commands—just like a computer.

In epilepsy and its related disorders, instead of firing when it is told, affected brain cells fire spontaneously on their own accord. This disturbs the balance in the brain and the surrounding cells get confused and also start firing. The result is a total electrical imbalance in a region of the brain or the whole brain itself. In some cases, the imbalance stays in a certain region, yielding focal symptoms such as staring or shaking one region of the body. In others, the imbalance spreads and the entire brain is affected, causing the classic "tonic-clonic" or "grand mal" seizure most of us are familiar with. This is the type of seizure that causes a person to shake violently, bite their tongue, urinate on themselves, and wake up confused. Most seizures last a minute or two, but occasionally, there can be a progression to a nonstop seizure called "status epilepticus," which is life threatening. Status can cause the body's temperature to rise, put extra stress on the heart, cause a buildup of acid in the blood and kidney, and restrict blood flow to the brain.

Other than status, why does shaking for a minute or two become so concerning? Obviously, quality of life is drastically affected: these patients cannot drive or perform work as usual; always in fear for when the next attack may occur. More importantly, these episodes restrict blood flow to the brain, essentially depriving the brain of its much-needed oxygen. Over time, these attacks can become longer and longer and cause irreversible brain damage—hence the reason modern medicine is so aggressive at preventing them. We treat epileptics with different classes of medications to help control and prevent their seizures. Once an appropriate regimen is found, most epileptics live normal lives and are seizure free for long periods of time.

## The Spirit

It was a warm day—about 80 percent humidity and a temperature of 85 degrees Fahrenheit. A warm Caribbean breeze would blow through every so often, and our fans and air-conditioning kept the air cool and well circulated in the ER. Every fifteen minutes or so, we would lose power, but the generators would start up a minute or two later, keeping the air moving. Astutely so, the ventilators were put on their own generator to continue working during power outages.

Even with constantly circulating air, I found myself sweating most of the time. As a matter of fact, I carried a handkerchief in my pocket to wipe my sweat every few minutes. I remember some of my prior trips to Haiti where during the warmer seasons we had days of 100 percent humidity and temperature measured 98 degrees Fahrenheit, which effectively felt like 110 degrees Fahrenheit. Having grown up in the Inland Empire of Southern California, I am used to dry heat. I could tolerate 110 degrees Fahrenheit or higher temperatures in dry heat. When it got too hot, I just hid under a tree or drenched my face with water. Humidity, however, is God's punishment to man. There is nowhere to hide from humidity. I was always in a state of sweat when in Haiti during the peak humid season. To keep things somewhat tolerable, I would tie a bandana around my forehead to keep the sweat out of my eyes. At one point, I was sweating so much that I was chafing my groin. Luckily, a fellow volunteer had baby powder, which saved the day. One volunteer from Michigan said it best "I think I'm melting in Haiti."

All in all today, I was pretty comfortable. My sweat gauge was fairly low—when my shirt pocket showed sweat lines, I knew it was bad— today it was still dry. It was about 1600 hours (4 in the afternoon) and my emergency room was under control. I had a patient with an asthma flare in my first bed that was doing pretty good after some breathing treatments, and I knew he would go home after another treatment or two. My second bed was empty, and I took a break while I could. I was pretty hungry, having missed lunch, and had been eyeing my Promax Cookies 'n Cream bar. No sooner had I grabbed and opened the bar than in came running one of my translators,

62                                                           *The Loa*

Pierre. Pierre is an odd character—tall, lanky, and he walks hunched forward. With his crossed eyes and jittery gait, he said, "We have a spirit attack coming in, Doc." I nearly split my pants—ironically, the translator who himself sometimes looked like he was possessed was frantic about a possession. At first I thought it was a joke and snickered, however, the expression on his face told me otherwise. He was serious.

In came Marie, a ten-year-old female still dressed in her Haitian school uniform. Haitian uniforms are of French descent; thus picture a white pressed shirt and plaid skirt. She was not responsive and was being carried in by someone who looked like her mother. Her mother looked flustered—her hair was half-braided and scruffy. She had obviously been working on it when she was called out. Like most Haitians living in this warm tropical environment, the mother had a very thin halter top on, barely held up by two spaghetti straps. Her skirt was wrinkled and unkempt, indicating she was in a rush to get her clothes on.

I began my initial assessment: heart sounded good, lungs were clear, pupils were reactive to light. She wasn't fully alert yet but was mumbling words and moving her arms and legs, so I knew the computer up top was still working. The rest of the team was busy at work putting in an IV and getting blood drawn. As I was examining Marie, I asked Pierre to ask what happened and translate for me. Her mother spoke: Marie was at school and started complaining of a headache to her teacher. A minute later, she collapsed and was shaking violently and foaming from the mouth. The teacher sent

Marie's friend to go and fetch her mother. The shaking lasted for about two minutes and subsided. Marie remained unconscious and a few minutes later had another seizure, which lasted a minute or so. Slowly she awoke over the next thirty minutes, at which time her mother had arrived. Her mother immediately put her in her vehicle and left for our hospital. As they neared the hospital, Marie was speaking but confused; she was in what we call a post-ictal state. Post-ictal state is the time shortly after a seizure where brain is basically rebooting itself. People may talk and look around but are incoherent and don't comprehend or remember what is going on. As Marie and her mother were coming up to the gate, Marie had another attack, and the security guards let them straight through. Pierre was at the gate and helped direct the mother to the ER.

After stabilizing Marie by having an IV placed and ensuring she was breathing on her own and not actively seizing, I had our pharmacist ready a phenytoin load. Phenytoin is a medication good at preventing seizures and is the first go to and most commonly used medication for seizure prevention. The nurses were getting ready to inject this medication when I pulled the mother aside to get more information. No, this had not happened before; no, she was not taking any medications; no, she was not drinking or doing any drugs; no, there was no family history of seizures; no, she had no other medical problems; yes, she was a healthy child. Through Pierre, she began telling me her story.

Last night she and her neighbor had a row, which turned out pretty messy. Both their families have chickens that they raise for food and eggs. Marie's family owns twelve hens and two cocks, which are kept in her yard. The neighbor owns a few hens and one cock. In Haiti, most people who are lucky enough to own a house share property with others. The neighbor's chickens often straggle over to Marie's yard, and thus far, their meetings have been calm and chicken friendly. Chickens are fairly docile animals and easy to farm. But to make chickens, you need a cock. Cocks, on the other hand, act as their name implies. Roosters tend to be feisty creatures and are very territorial. They fight hard to keep their hens in line and dominate the roost. Both chicken families lived in peace and prosperity, minding their own business and occasionally bumping into one another. Yesterday, however, their meeting was not congenial.

Marie's mother was cooking dinner in the evening when she heard yelling. Curiously, she stepped outside to find her neighbor yelling at Marie. Apparently, Marie had not closed the fence to the roost and their cock had escaped. He nonchalantly meandered over to the neighbor's area where her cock was also out, patrolling his territory. When the two cocks saw each other, it was as if Edward Cullen and Jacob Black from the *Twilight Saga* were personified. What ensued next was nothing less than a gruesome battle for Bella—I mean, the hens and their territory—which eventually led to the death of the neighbor's cock. Enraged, the neighbor began screaming at Marie for her incompetence, and at this point Marie's mother walked in.

Marie's mother tried to calm the neighbor with no success. This was her favorite cock that had bred all her hens. She needed him to breed through the rest of the season. How was she going to get her eggs and next generation of chickens? Where would she get the money to buy another cock? Why didn't Marie just close the gate like she should have? Irate, the neighbor took possession of her prized rooster's corpse and stormed back to her house. Marie's mother could hear muffled voices, which sounded fairly emotional and angry. She thought nothing of it though and collected Marie and came back in to the house. She told Marie to avoid the neighbor until this was figured out and to be more careful next time. She then returned to cooking dinner and thought she would have to deal with this at a later time.

Looking back at the situation, Marie's mother now thought that the mumbling and sounds she heard coming from the neighbor's house were the cause of the current situation. She believed the neighbor cast a spell or curse on Marie. She felt she never could trust the neighbor and that she had come from a lower class family who they all tried to avoid. It was quite possible, in her mother's view, that the neighbor cursed them. All that rattling and noise was "she putting bad spell on us." This bad spell was a spirit that her neighbor called upon for retaliation. "She called a spirit to attack my baby," translated Pierre. Pierre was convinced that Marie's mother's story was true and this was the result of a curse. He proceeded to tell me that Voudou is very common in Haiti and things like this happen all the time.

## Voudou

Voudou (misnomer Voodoo) is an ancient religion of the African peoples. It is thought to have started over 7,500 years ago, making it one of the oldest religions in the world. Voudou was the main belief system of many African tribes and is still practiced in parts of Africa. During the slave trade, African slaves took their belief with them and it evolved with time, becoming Voodoo of Louisiana and Santeria of Cuba and the Bahamas. In Haitian Voudou there is a supreme god called Bondyи, derived from the French words *bon dieu*, "good god." Bondyи is the boss god. He rules over all others and is the creator of all. For the most part, he does not follow or involve himself with the daily lives of humans. He is busy with the happenings of the other gods (Loa) and their drama. Loas are lesser gods, subservient to Bondyи. They have their own life, which they live in their spiritual realm. They marry, have children, fight, and have temperaments just like humans. Loas interact directly with humans, and it is to Loas that people routinely pray, not to Bondyи, given his indifference to daily events.

Just as there are calm and brash tempered humans, there are varying levels of personality among the Loas. The calmer, more peaceful Loas are called cool Loas, while the angrier, violent Loas are considered warm. The drama among Loas is very similar to that among the gods in Greek mythology or deities in Hinduism. They fight, make love, and make war against each other. When praying to a Loa, if one desires good, one usually prays to a cool Loa. If one desires black magic and curses, one could incite the services of a warm Loa. For the most part, Voudou is a religion like any other—holding itself to strong ethical values of family, trust, sharing, and honesty. Just as in any culture, some choose to disregard these morals and are swayed by selfish and "evil" thoughts and motivations. This minority has been modeled in media as "Voodoo shaman," hence the reason a common person's description of Voudou always begins with a "Voodoo doll." In reality, Voodoo dolls are a type of *pwen*, or power object. These objects have some link to the desired person and are used to bring happiness, fortune, and health or the opposite: sadness, poverty, and sickness. Very few people practice this type of Voudou, and even fewer yet lay curses on others.

With the slave trade, Voudou was spread throughout the New World, including the Caribbean and parts of the United States such as Louisiana. At the height of the slave trade in the sixteenth century, traders worked hard to eliminate Voudou. Since most slave traders/owners were of monotheistic Anglican Christian descent, they despised Voudou for its polytheism. Through syncretism (combing of beliefs), the African slaves hid Voudou under the guise of conversion to Roman Catholicism and other Christian denominations. In order to keep their religion alive, believers and shamans likened Bondyи to the omniscient Judeo-Christian-Islamic God. Loas are no longer gods, however, but rather take on the role of saints. The slaves would thus be praying to one god but would seek guidance from saints (Loa). In this way, their cultural heritage and religion was still propagated. Over time, the concept of Loa as saints solidified to the point that now almost all Haitians believe in the monotheistic god of the Catholics and see the Loas truly as saints.

When in need of help or guidance, the Haitians will perform Voudou ceremonies in which they call upon the Loas for assistance. This is done by a shaman or elder who recites prayers (usually starting with Hail Mary) and starts a chant or song. Others may then join in and the singing (sometimes accompanied by a ritualistic sacrifice of a chicken or pig) invites the Loas to Earth. When they arrive, they take possession of the singer or another member and speak and act through them. When possession is completed, the Loas leave and the ceremony is over. Not all ceremonies ask for the Loas to come in spirit; most are simply asking for guidance or assistance.

I recall walking into the pediatric tent of the old hospital one day to find a Voudou ritual underway. A patient was gravely ill with a poor prognosis and the medical team decided to withdraw medical care the next day, essentially turning off the machine that was breathing for the child. The child was deemed brain-dead at that point, so the family asked a priest for help. The Voudou priest was singing, and most of the Haitians in the tent (other patients and their families) chanted along. He was singing for one of the Loas to come and save this child the next morning, and if the child was not to be saved, then to guide the child safely to the underworld. I was told that the priest needed to sacrifice a chicken to complete the ceremony, and this was done later that night outside the hospital premises.

The next morning the child died.

## Spirit-o-gram

To best determine what type of seizures a person has, we perform an EEG (electroencephalogram). This test requires hooking up leads on numerous regions of the head to monitor the electrical activity of the brain. A neurologist then reads this activity and determines what type of seizure disorder a patient has and often what part of the brain the seizure originates from and affects. Based on the type of seizure, a tailored medication regimen is created for the patient. Knowing Marie needed a more extensive workup I thought, *How am I supposed to explain all of this to someone who does not understand Western medicine, is uneducated, and most importantly, believes this is a spirit attack?*

I pride myself on my ability to explain complex medical concepts in simple, easy-to-understand terms. My patients back home in the United States always thank me for explaining their diseases so clearly to them. I often hear, "I never understood this disease before." I began to think basics: *Maybe I should start by explaining how cells use electricity to talk. Then I could expand on what a seizure really is and how it needs to be treated. She'd understand that, right?* At that point, it hit me: where in all of this did the spirit come in? After hearing the mother's story, I knew she was convinced this was a spirit attack, and a ten-minute interaction with some foreign doctor with a funny moustache was *not* going to change the beliefs she developed over a lifetime. Instead, I had to compromise. I would continue to treat this as a spirit attack but integrate a few western ideas. I told the mother that Marie had been with me for about an hour now and her blood work came back negative. No signs of an infection or organ damage, no malaria, no typhoid. I informed the mother that although we knew Marie was attacked by spirits, we did not know which spirit it was. Was it the malaria spirit gone undiagnosed (which happens often)? Was it an epilepsy spirit? A brain tumor spirit? We needed to find out which spirit it was and for that we needed an EEG. I called it a spirit-o-gram (-gram being Latin for drawing), essentially a drawing of the spirit or way to identify which spirit was plaguing Marie. The medication I gave Marie would help keep the spirits at bay for now, but we needed to determine the etiology of her seizures to best treat them. The mother acknowledged and accepted my explanation.

Once Marie was stabilized, given a medication to prevent further seizures, awake, and talking, it was time to send her to get a spirit-o-gram. Our hospital, albeit fairly well equipped, does not have access to an EEG, let alone a neurologist to interpret the test. The closest place that would accept Marie without an exorbitant amount of cash was the General Hospital. The General is the state-run public hospital. Since majority of Haitians cannot afford medical care, they brave their luck waiting in long lines at the General to be seen. The General is staffed by local Haitian doctors, and occasionally, foreign doctors would come in and assist. On one of my prior trips, I was sent to the General a few times to help take care of their patients in the intensive care unit (ICU) and assist in the outpatient clinic. When I arrived, no doctor had visited the ICU for two days. The patients were a mess. Some had not been on any medications for a day; others had wound infections that hadn't been cleaned for days. After stabilizing the ICU patients, I would help out in the clinic.

The General was seeing over five hundred patients a day in their outpatient clinic. Their examining area consisted of a small coffee table separating two chairs, one for me and one for my patient. Five of these makeshift stations were thrown together inside a small-sized disaster response tent, much like a circus tent. For almost a quarter mile outside the tent, there was the line of people waiting to be seen. The days I spent there, I would see 125 patients daily. Privacy was a joke. At one point, I had to examine the testicles of a gentleman complaining of swelling, and as I was inquiring where we could go, he stood up, lowered his pants, and showed me his testicles. I was pretty surprised at first, but on second thought, I realized these people were living in such densely populated tent cities in poverty that privacy was a luxury, not a necessity.

Having seen and worked at the General Hospital, I knew why patients despised going there. I thought it was going to be an uphill battle convincing the mother to take Marie there for an EEG. To my surprise, it was the opposite. After my showing understanding and cultural competence by acknowledging the spirit attacks, the mother was quite cooperative. Of course I did not tell the mother they were going to get an EEG; rather I told her Marie needed a spirit-o-gram and a spirit photograph (CT Scan imaging of the brain) to determine which spirit was causing this. Through Pierre, she voiced her understanding and gratitude for the care Marie had received in our hospital.

Marie was awake at this point and responsive. She giggled when I played with her hair and moved all of her extremities. She looked fairly stable and showed no signs of permanent brain damage. I proceeded to complete the necessary paperwork and gave the referral to the mother. She gathered her belongings, scooted up a smiling Marie, and they were off. As she walked out the door, through Pierre she said, "Thank you, I will go to the General to find out which Loa is attacking my Marie." With a touch of cultural competency and appropriate initial medical assessment and care, Marie was stabilized and sent to the General Hospital.

Two days later Marie and mother returned to tell me the spirit photograph showed nothing (meaning a normal head CT scan) and the spirit-o-gram (EEG) said Marie had "the epilepsy Loa." Marie was given medications and her mother wanted me to approve of them before they were continued. Marie was given phenytoin and sent home, and I told mother this was a great medication and agreed with its use for this Loa. In an interesting marriage of western allopathic medicine with traditional Voudou belief, Marie was treated appropriately without disrespectfully ignoring the family's beliefs, leading to a great outcome everyone was happy with – a seizure free Marie.

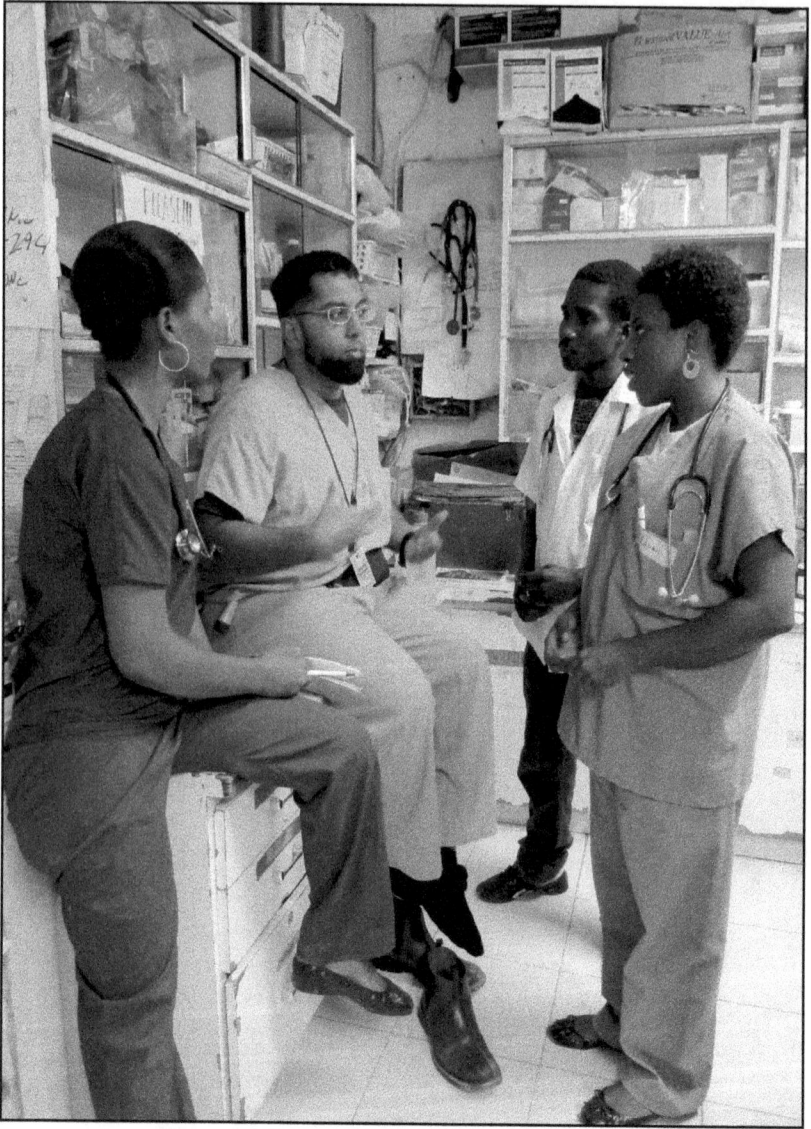

Case discussion with Haitian doctors in training. Teaching and sharing of knowledge is an integral part of successful international medical missions.

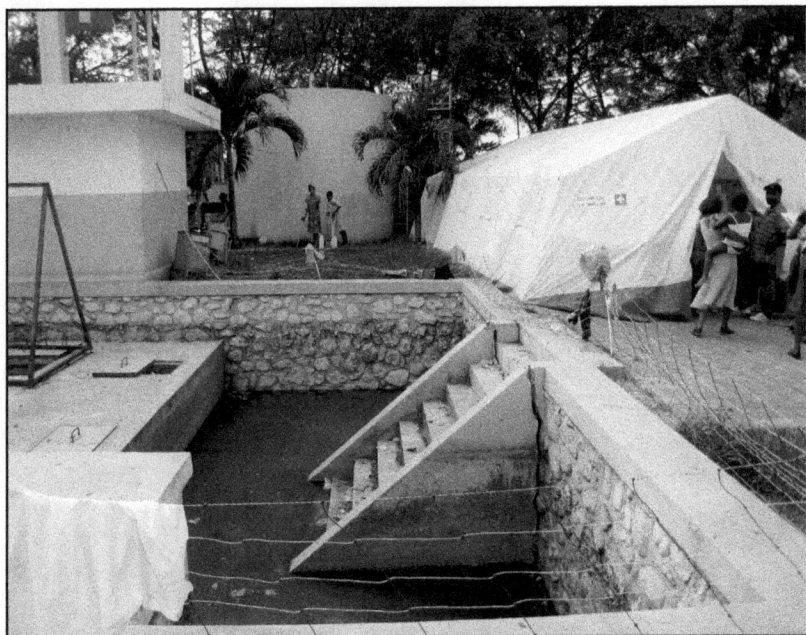

Pediatric ward tent on the grounds of the General Hospital. Note the cesspool of water breeding mosquitoes next to the tent.

# Common Things Being Common

*Our greatest glory is not in never falling, but in rising every time we fall.*

- Confucius -

# Cyanotic baby

Given the less than ideal resources, part of practicing medicine in Haiti requires identifying early warning signs rather than waiting until a patient decompensates. One night in the ER a woman brought her newly born nephew to be evaluated. He was born 3 hours ago and never quite had a good skin color per the aunt. He had a slightly blue hue to him and she was concerned that this was not normal.

A blue (cyanotic) newborn is concerning. Infants with certain congenital heart defects will grow appropriately in the womb since oxygenation of blood is done by the placenta. When these children are born their heart lesions (cyanotic lesions) become apparent as used blood does not get re-oxygenated as it should, causing the babies to have a blue hue. These lesions can vary from emergent life threatening conditions to those which require urgent but non-emergent surgical intervention.

The baby did have a slight bluish hue to him but nothing that was out of the ordinary. There are some babies who take longer than others to really gain good skin color after birth. We checked the baby's oxygen saturation and found it to be in the lower normal range. In a clinical setting, as long as the baby was feeding I would let the baby go home and have the family keep a close eye. I may even consider ordering imaging studies such as an ultrasound of the heart. Here, however, if the baby did have a true cyanotic lesion it may not be easy for the family to bring the baby back. Ordering an ultrasound was also a difficult process. Even if ordered, it may take a day or two for a radiologist to interpret the reading, which may be too late. So I decided to watch the baby in the ER for a few hours. Baby ate well and never dropped his oxygen saturation below an acceptable limit.

In my own comfort zone back home this baby would have been sent back home after a bit or parental reassuring. In Haiti I knew access to care was a problem and thus even second guessed my clinical assessment. Scared that I would send a potentially sick baby home I kept them in my ER for hours (more than anything to make myself feel better about sending them home). Had there been a true lesion there's not much that would have been done either way. There was no pediatric cardiac surgeon to be found in all of PaP.

What would have been a fairly common assessment back home scared the living daylights out of me in Haiti. Not having the access to specialists and exams I was used to really shook my confidence and made me practice more conservatively when I was in Haiti.

---

We physicians are trained investigators. We are faced with a set of complaints, array of physical findings (and often lack thereof), and lab results/images to sift through. In the end, the job revolves around problem solving - identify the possibilities, narrow them down to the most likely cause(s), and provide the appropriate remedy. While trying to identify the cause(s) of a particular ailment, the well trained sleuth recites the mantra taught in medical schools around the world: "common things are common." Meaning, as we become academically perplexed by the array of medical possibilities, we must not lose sight of the common etiologies of disease. I once had an eager junior medical student tell me he thought he had diagnosed a case of neuro-syphilis. The patient was a young man who had been admitted for confusion and altered mental status. He had a history of promiscuity so the student thought it must have been syphilis infecting the brain - something he had just studied about a few weeks ago. Blood work and time would show that the patient had actually overdosed on Lysergic Acid Diethylamide (LSD, or the street drug Acid). After sobering up for a few hours the patient walked out of the hospital. I told the student what was once told to me, a modified version of the phrase coined by the late Dr. Theodore Woodward: "When you hear hoof beats behind you, don't expect to see a zebra unless you're in Africa or the Zoo."

A few months after the earthquake, while still in the tent hospital, I was presented with a middle aged man for admission, Roger. The ER physician who had seen him was worried about a severe penile infection. During my evaluation I asked the patient numerous times about the relevant history. Every time he stuck with the same story: The penis began appearing red about 2 weeks prior and quickly progressed to the state it was in today. After confirming he had no other medical problems, I covered him with a robe and slowly advanced to exam the penis.

There was no privacy in the tent – cots on all sides filled with patients and family members. Knowing this, I planned to take my time during the exam to ensure some level of modesty. As I began to slowly lift a part of the robe to steal a glance, Roger grabbed the robe and pulled it off, brashly revealing his entire member for all around to see. Modesty, it seemed, was not a concern for Roger. I would learn later that modesty is a cultural definition and modesty in the humid stale heat of the Caribbean is *very* different then modesty in the U.S. Women routinely remove their shirts in public to poor water on their chest, breast feed, or to change shirts. It was bad enough already that we were in practically a giant circus tent and now we were going to be the main act. To my surprise, not one person around me cared that Roger had disrobed and no one seemed to be looking. They imparted him with an almost invisible veil of privacy, ignoring everything that was occurring. Surprised but reassured that I wasn't the main act, I proceeded to perform my examination.

Examining a patient who is disrobed is quite an intimate act. Voluntary disrobing is something reserved usually for two groups of people; those we love, and those who take care of our health. As a physician, examining the naked human body is much like listening to a story book. What may be a caress from a lover across the chest is a blunt palpation of bony landmarks by the physician. The small recess of privacy, which is modesty, we are allowed to enter and freely explore. Allowed to touch, feel, smell, and use all our senses to understand the body, we listen to the story the body has to tell us. We listen to the heart beat, breath flowing to and from the lungs; we feel the state of the skin; we smell the odors; and we watch the subtle rise and fall of the chest. Using all of our senses, we take in the person in front of us, combine their findings with analytical knowledge

*Common Things Being Common*

obtained through years of education and arrive at a diagnosis and plan to help alleviate said ailment. A common saying in medicine goes: "a good doctor can diagnose 80% of ailments by history and physical exam alone." The entire process is quite personal and is an art perfected by years of studying and practice in small personal settings. To lose that patient-provider intimacy by having Roger expose himself in front of complete strangers was a bit intimidating. Nonetheless, I had to proceed with my exam.

Roger now fully disrobed, his sickness was obvious. He was cachectic and emaciated – I could see all his ribs through his paper thin skin. I felt around the groin area and palpated multiple small hard nodules. These were his lymph nodes which were quite enlarged. It was immediately obvious that Roger either had a very severe infection, HIV, TB, or cancer. Looking down, my eyes befell his member and I gasped. About 3 centimeters from the base of the shaft, the penis had a discoloration which can only be described as deathly. A gnarly purple ulcer was eating away at the shaft, and the head of the penis was nowhere to be found. The ulcer had completely eroded away the head of the penis leaving an amalgam of tissue, melted and blended into an eerie imitation of what a penis should look like. It looked like someone had set the head of his penis on fire and allowed it to reform, like a melted birthday candle. Surprisingly Roger had no pain in the penis or any sensation at all from where the ulcer started, to the end of the penis. My poking and prodding elicited no response from Roger. Out came white, yellow, and red fluid. A mix of purulent, foul smelling liquid and blood seeped from the ulcer, which circumferentially engulfed his man part. One diagnosis from medical school came to mind, Fournier Gangrene.

Fournier Gangrene is a form of necrotizing fasciitis, referred to in the media as the "flesh eating bacteria." It is a highly aggressive infection of the male genitalia by normally co-existent bacteria that run amuck. Often, it is seen in light of an immunocompromising disease such as diabetes or HIV and spreads rapidly – in hours to days in some cases. Rare, the disease has been reported 600 times in the literature since its identification in 1883 through 1996. Treatment involves early identification and aggressive antibiotic therapy. Surgical debridement of the wound is an organ and life saving measure. Identification of the causative organism is crucial to allow microbial directed therapy, specifically targeting the culprit. If not identified and treated early, the infection can spread throughout the body and lead to death in days.

I had never seen Fournier Gangrene in my career but the severity of the ulceration and timeframe Roger swore by concerned me. I started him on antibiotics and immediately found the general surgeon. The general surgeon, another U.S. volunteer, took one look at the penis and agreed with my assessment. When asked about wound debridement, she said he would likely need an amputation of his penis. She would have to remove most of the penis, leaving only a small nub for urination. This was a surgery she did not feel fully competent in and preferred an urologist to be present for the procedure to lend their expertise.

We had no urologist on our volunteer team and thus had to call for a Haitian urologist. After making multiple phone calls we were told the urologist would come by that night to assess the situation. This same urologist had been consulted on other patients over the past few weeks. He had been dubbed "The Batman Doctor" or "BatDoc" by us. He came at random hours during the day or night. Without finding the working physician, he came, evaluated the patient, sometimes wrote a note with his recommendations and disappeared like Batman. Sometimes he would not even leave a note, just disappear as fast as he had appeared. The only reason we knew he had come would be because a nurse or the patient would tell us. When he left a note in the chart, it was scribbled in illegible French and when he didn't, we had to ask the patients what he had said. Coming from the patient, half the time they didn't know what he was talking about or what his recommendation was. Bat Doc was called in for this patient and who knew when he would make an appearance. I knew I would have to keep an eye out for him to ensure the surgery was done in a timely fashion.

Bag after bag of antibiotics were run and two days had gone by without any sign of Bat Doc. Roger was stable and the infection seemed to have slowed a bit. He was still quite sick and any small insult such as a cold or dehydration could be enough to tip him over the edge into a downward spiral. I called for the urologist numerous times only to be told that he would come in a few hours each time. A few hours came and went over and over again. It was 2 A.M. and I was the on call doctor for the night. Rounding on the patient the next cot over, I saw someone approach Roger and start looking through the chart. Finally, there days later, Bat Doc appeared. I approached him and described the situation.

Bat Doc muttered a few words in Creole to Roger which sounded like he was confirming the chain of events. With a sense of urgency, he pulled down Roger's blanket and examined the disease. Sternly, he asked Roger a few more questions in Creole. Unsatisfied with the answer, he slapped Roger across the face and asked the question again. The slap wasn't a soft encouraging tap, but rather a paternal like stern motivation of a slap for a new answer. It was the kind of slap you get from mom after she knows you've lied to her; the kind of slap you tell the truth after. Roger immediately answered – and to my surprise he spoke for about two minutes. When he was done, taken aback, I didn't know what to do. Should I stop Bat Doc; restrain him; ask him to leave? I had never imagined a doctor being violent towards a patient let alone ever seen it done. I was fed up – first off, it had taken Bat Doc three days to respond to an urgent call and now he had overstepped a fundamental boundary in the patient-physician relationship.

As I readied myself to ask him to leave, Bat Doc opened his mouth and uttered something that took me by surprise. "As you say in the States, this is not a Zebra, it is a Horse," Bat Doc said. Confused, I asked him to expand. Apparently the slap across the face helped Roger get his story straight. All of a sudden the chain of events came back clearly to Roger – this disease started with a small ulceration about seven months ago, not a few days as he had told us. Over the course of months he had been losing weight and the ulcer had developed into what it is today. The ulcer had actually looked about the same for the past four weeks. The discharge had started about three weeks ago and slowly progressed. He had been evaluated by

*Common Things Being Common*

a Haitian doctor already and given the diagnosis of penile cancer. Roger ignored the Haitian doctor and came to our hospital with a new story hoping for better care. Bat Doc told me he was sure this was penile cancer and not Fournier Gangrene. He had seen Fournier Gangrene multiple times and was positive this was not it. This was penile cancer, plain and simple. The pus and discharge was from a secondary infection of the cancerous tissue. After finding multiple nodules on prostate exam Bat Doc determined the disease had spread and did not warrant surgical treatment. Later that day I obtained a chest radiograph which confirmed Bat Doc's assessment: there were cancer nodules on the x-ray. Roger was given a terminal diagnosis of metastatic penile cancer and was to be discharged home the next day with oral antibiotics.

The next day I talked with Roger more and asked him why he had not told me the truth. Roger said he knew that if he told the truth we would have not admitted him. He knew this was a chronic condition that he would die from soon but did what he had done to be admitted and evaluated by "The American Doctors" for one last hope of cure. Now that we had arrived at the same conclusion a Haitian physician had already told him weeks prior, he was satisfied going home to die. I apologized for not being able to help him, gave him $200 US dollars for end of life expenses and discharged him later that day. What leftover funds I had from my donations I made a point to give to patients in need. Each trip I usually had around $1000 cash left over that I would distribute. Roger went home; satisfied he had been seen by "The American Doctors." All along, the Haitian doctors he had been seeing had provided accurate diagnoses and in the end, corrected "The American Doctors." And I finally had a sighting of the infamous Bat Doc.

Later, I asked Bat Doc if he had ever reported the Fournier Gangrene cases he had seen, that there were only 600 or so cases reported in the literature. His response to me was humbly, "If I said I saw a Zebra in Haiti, no one would believe me." With no powerhouse academic institution providing him with administration time to work on scholarly projects or lending its name to his paper, getting published would be an insurmountable task. I understood his situation and thanked him for his time – Bat Doc reminded me that hoof beats even in Haiti are probably from horses, not zebras.

## Tomas

At times, when we had enough volunteers, we were sent to neighboring clinics to help see patients. One day I was working at a clinic near the capitol building. The clinic was housed in the police station and originally called the "Police Clinic." That day Tomas, a homeless twelve year old boy, walked in holding his right hand in a blood soaked rag. He spoke some broken English and told me he had cut his finger. As many homeless children do, he cleaned the wheels of cars stopped at intersections for whatever pennies the drivers would throw at them. When cleaning one of the wheels he sliced the distal tip of his index finger (the pointer finger) on a protruding piece of metal. It bled significantly and he covered it with a rag and ran over a block to this clinic.

After anesthetizing his finger I cleaned it thoroughly and found that

*Common Things Being Common*

he had nearly cut off the tip of his finger. It was hanging on by a few strands of muscle fibers and skin beneath the nail. Although gruesome looking, the wound itself was fairly easy to sew together. Luckily his bone wasn't exposed and the wound edges were even. Exposed bone is dangerous as it can become infected and requires a more thorough procedure involving amputation of the distal tip and a flap of skin sewn over the bone to protect it. After thoroughly washing it out, I sewed the tip back on and wrapped his finger. During the entire procedure, he hadn't shown any pain. He didn't move when I injected lidocaine to numb the finger. He didn't groan as the lidocaine burned before making his finger numb. He had the maturity and pain threshold many adults don't even possess. Impressed, I complimented him on his steadfastness as I gave him his prophylactic tetanus vaccination (given anytime there is a wound involving metal to prevent tetanus if the patient is due for a booster). While I was writing a prescription for antibiotics, Tomas suddenly broke down in tears.

Out of nowhere he began sobbing heavily. Before I could even ask what was bothering him he opened up to me. Prior to the earthquake Tomas lived in an average neighborhood with his little brother, Pierre, who was 6 years old at the time, mother, and father. He was 10 years old and enjoyed life. Mother would wake him up in the morning; make him a breakfast of beans and rice to go along with fresh orange juice. After his energizing meal he would be shooed off to school with his brother. "I wanted to be a doctor," he would say. After school he would come home and spend the next few hours outside playing soccer or other activities with his neighborhood friends. At the end of the day dinner with the family followed by group television time concluded the evening. Life was simple; life was secure - he was a happy child.

On January 12, 2010 his life changed. When the earthquake struck he was in his home on the first floor with Pierre. They were watching American cartoons dubbed in French on the television when the shaking began. Mom and Dad were both upstairs. Tomas thought nothing of the shaking at first - it took a lot to pull his attention from old episodes of Looney Toons. A few seconds later things began falling off the shelves and he knew something scary was happening. He tried running upstairs to find his parents but did not make it. The staircase shook violently and the first 3 steps disintegrated in front of his eyes. Scared, Tomas grabbed Pierre and ran outside. A neighboring family took a hold of the two of them and ran towards the middle of the road. Pierre screamed for his parents and Tomas tried to calm him down.

As the Earth continued to rumble, the weak man-made abodes were stressed to their limits. The diluted concrete and smooth re-bars, shortcuts for saving money in construction costs, were unable to bear the stress. Tomas and Pierre watched, horrified. "Like a toy," Tomas described the house as it swayed side to side and finally gave way. Like a boxer receiving the final knockout punch, the pillars holding the house up buckled and the top of the house came roaring down. A large cloud of dust overtook the group and they panicked. Tomas lost hold of Pierre and ran about trying to find him. In the dust, Tomas could hear screaming, running, and the sound of other buildings falling. The dust enveloped him and he began coughing. He stood still to wait for the dust to clear, unsure what was going on.

A few minutes later the dust began to settle and a figure was making its way over to him. As it neared, the silhouette of a human slowly transformed into that of a specter. A woman walked towards him - completely white and eerie, he thought it was a ghost. As it neared he finally recognized her as his neighbor covered in dust so only her teeth and the white of her eyes were visible. More and more people came into view as the dust fell to the ground. He realized these weren't ghosts, but rather his neighbors covered by dust. Behind one group he spotted his brother and rushed to embrace him. Together, they saw what was left of their home - a pile of twisted metal and powdered concrete. Mom and dad never left the building. In seconds of shaking Tomas went from being a happy child to an orphan.

The next few days the boys lived with the neighbors on the street. They were later relocated to an orphanage but found it less than ideal. Food was scarce, bullying was common, and the people running the orphanage often resorted to physical violence to keep children in line. During meal time, he was always bullied by older kids who took his food from him. He would have to share Pierre's food and they both went hungry every day. Two weeks into their stay, Tomas was fed up and eloped with Pierre. Since then he had been living on the street with a family he knew prior to the earthquake. They provided some level of security but Tomas had to earn his own money and food. To make money he had done multiple tasks from washing cars to shining shoes. Recently, he began cleaning car wheels.

With the little money he made during the day, Tomas bought food for his brother and him. Tomas sobbed as he told his story, tears flowing from between his fingers which held his face tightly. "If my mother was still alive I wouldn't be here," he cried. "She always took care of me and Pierre. I miss her." My eyes began to well up with tears and I didn't know what I could do to help him. I had done what I was trained to, fix a medical ailment. The bigger problem at hand, however, I was not able to fix. I held Tomas in my arms and let him cry into my shoulders. When he was done he gathered his belongings and was getting ready to leave. I handed him some cash for food for Pierre and himself. As he left he said, "My mother would never let this happen to me, but she would have liked you." In those few minutes, I felt closer to Tomas than many of the thousands of patients I had treated back home. What would have been a common laceration repair elsewhere turned into anything but – it became one of the most touching moments of my life.

At the tender age of 12, most of us can fondly remember a care free world. One in which we played when we wanted, ate when we needed, and did as we pleased. We didn't worry about having to bring food home or find a safe place to sleep for the night. We were just kids. However, around the world at the age of 12 children are forced to take on the roles of adults. Many go to war, work, and even get married. Maturity is a socially derived concept, true, but it also has a biological basis. Twelve is a young age no matter what society one is raised in. Even though many 12 year olds may be starting families of their own, they have a tremendous (and often overbearing) support system to help guide them through. At 12, Tomas was a kid forced to act like an adult responsible for his brother Pierre. Without his guidance and leadership, they both could have died by now. I can remember at the age of 12 I was in junior high school; confused and unsure of myself, I gave my parents a hard time. I argued about everything I could; from the way I dressed to the friends I hung out with to how I combed my hair. Here was Tomas, at the age of 12, not only showing an amazing amount of maturity but basically leading his family and keeping Pierre alive. What started as a simple cut to the finger of a kid became more; it was a threat to the livelihood of the bread earner of the family.

---

Sometimes common things are all too common and become confusing. In Haiti, a common complaint in the ER is *Mwen gen tèt fè mal*, meaning *I have a headache* or *my head aches*. Culturally, it is a way of stating that overall one isn't feeling well or maybe fatigued. Often the symptoms would be described as, "my heart hurts, my stomach hurts, and my head aches." These vague complaints are often attributed to conditions such as insomnia, seasonal allergies, and depression – common ailments which plague this ravished country.

Especially concerning are finding these vague symptoms in children. A child complaining of stomach ache or general *tèt fè mal* was often due to a parasitic infection. Given the lack of clean water and food, many children were chronic carriers of parasites. The most common parasitic infection in children is infestation of worms, or nematodes. The phylum of Nematoda, also known as ringworms, has over 500,000 species. Another common worm is the Cestoda (tapeworm), from the phylum Platyhelminthes. A few of the common worms that infect humans include pinworms, echinococcus, whipworm, Ascaris and hookworms. Worms can consume up to 20% of a person's food. In a situation where food intake is already minimal, 20% becomes a significant loss of much needed calories.

The World Health Organization estimates that intestinal parasites infect more than a third of the entire world's population, most of which live in developing nations. Many de-worming campaigns have been started to help alleviate the problem. Since the worm life cycle includes infected and uninfected humans and animals, eradicating the disease is a complex process. General population intervention is the most efficient eradication strategy. An entire city will be 'de-wormed' by giving Albendazole or a similar medication to all inhabitants, especially children who are at higher risk to acquire, have, and spread worms. Any individual, especially children, who complain of fatigue symptoms, weight loss, vague abdominal pain, or look like they are infected with worms received a treatment of Albendazole. A simple and effective regimen, a onetime dose was adequate for most types of worm infections.

When a child presented to the ER with vague abdominal or generalized symptoms, we always gave them a dose of an anti-parasitic agent. If nothing else, it was a form of "herd immunity" – in which to protect the entire population (herd) we treated everyone we could. Our hospital and many other organizations working in Haiti organized massive city wide treatment projects in which we travelled to a community and "de-wormed" the whole group by providing medication to everyone at once.

During one of these excursions to a local tent city a mother brought her child, Dante, to be evaluated. Dante was seven years old but looked like he was four. His head was far too large for his body, making him look slightly alien like. His body was skin and bones. His eyes seem to bulge out of his skull. Chronically malnourished, he showed signs of having been this way for some time. He was drastically short for his age and wore a loose t-shirt and shorts. His arms and legs were skinny but his feet were swollen. His abdomen was large and looked obese to the untrained eye. I, however, had seen abdomens like this hundreds of times, but in adults.

The abdomen was that of a typical adult patient with liver cirrhosis I have cared for numerous times back home. In these patients, the liver slowly shuts down for different reasons (alcohol mostly but sometimes from infection) and fails to make the protein albumin. Albumin is a protein that circulates through the body in the blood stream. Protein draws water to it, much like a sponge. When the body lacks protein such as albumin, the fluid in blood has no reason to stay in the blood vessels and seeps out into the surrounding tissue, causing edema and ascites. Ascites is fluid which ends up in the abdomen where it shouldn't be. Dante's abdomen had ascites and edema – he was low on protein.

Mother told me that Dante had been losing weight drastically over the past two years. Access to food was difficult and they ate once every day or other day at most. Over the past year, Dante began slowing down in his mental development as well. She said he began forgetting things such as the alphabet and how to count. More recently, he seemed to be aggravated all the time and would cry for every little thing and just didn't seem himself to her.

Given Dante's appearance and the history of weight loss with difficulty accessing food, it was obvious he was suffering from severe malnutrition. More concerning were the behavioral changes and memory loss and swelling of the abdomen and feet. I was concerned he had acquired a malnutrition syndrome called Kwashiorkor. Kwashiorkor is a syndrome of severe malnutrition in which the body is faced with protein and vitamin deficiency which leads to a severely catabolic state. Energy use in the body is defined as being either anabolic or catabolic. Anabolic builds up (like anabolic steroids) and catabolic breaks down. Normally, the body has a balance between the two. In Kwashiorkor, the body is spending more energy daily then it is getting from food, leading to an overall catabolic state. The body breaks down its own muscles for nutrients leading to a severe protein deficient state. Without adequate nutrition, the body stops growing and the brain stops developing. Hair thins, teeth fall out, the body stops growing and with time, permanent neurological damage occurs, leading to mental retardation and eventually death. Treatment involves providing adequate nutrition. Protein has to be slowly reintroduced into the diet to prevent complications of re-feeding

I wasn't sure if intestinal parasites could cause such severe malnutrition but decided a prolonged course of an anti-parasitic agent was a reasonable first step along with multi-vitamin tablets. We prepared a bag of medications for Dante and handed it to mother, explaining how the pills were to be taken. I asked mom what was happening to the food aid being delivered by international organizations to the tent cities and she said she rarely received it. Turns out the tent cities had their own complex crime system and a few gangs of thugs ran the show. All delivered aid was picked through according to social rank. Police officers got first dibs, taking home whatever they wanted for their families or more often, to sell the aid in the black market which was now prominent in Haiti. Local thugs took what they wanted next, followed by their friends and so forth. By the time it was the average Haitian's turn, there was little to nothing left. Thus Dante and his family ate only when they were able to earn enough money from begging and even then, very little.

Dante was in a catabolic state when he really needed to be in an anabolic growing state, and the cure for his ailment first and foremost was access to a constant food supply. I recommended to mother that she take Dante to the pediatric hospital and they would likely admit him for treatment and nutrition - she said she would consider it. She was fed up and disillusioned with Haitian medical care having been to numerous doctors and hospitals in the past only to be sent home each time with a handful of pills of some sort. I assured her that with Dante in the condition he was now, the pediatric hospital would admit him. She seemed reassured with this and agreed to take him. I gave my lunch I had brought with me to Dante and his medications to his mother. Dante smiled and said Mêci (thank you).

I remember learning about Kwashiorkor in medical school as being a relatively common disease in certain regions of the world where access to food was limited, such as sub-Saharan Africa and India. I never saw the disease back home and never expected to see it during my career. Yet here I was, hours away from home and familiarity in a new culture diagnosing something I had learned about in fleeting in a medical school thousands of miles away. It finally made sense why we were forced to memorize so much in medical school – one never knew when we may use it. What would be seen as a Zebra back home, ironically was a Horse here in Haiti. I prayed Dante would be seen in the pediatric hospital and what I said about him being admitted would hold true. I knew there was a chance the hospital may not admit him since mom had no way to pay but I couldn't get myself to say this to her. Instead, I gave her $100 and told her to use this to pay for any costs that may hold him from treatment. I don't know what ever happened to Dante but with appropriate caloric repletion there was a good chance he would do well. It was unclear if this cognitive delay was too far advanced to recover but children are resilient – and with this hope I leave the story of Dante.

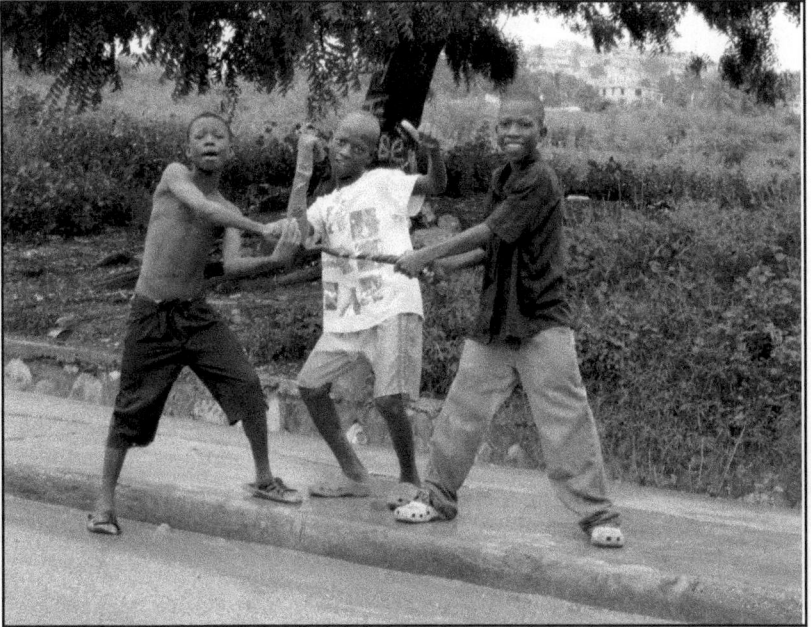

Homeless children on the streets of PaP playing while waiting for cars to stop. When a vehicle stops, the kids run out into the road to shine the wheels and clean the car for pennies.

# Balrog

*If it is a terrifying thought that life is at the mercy of the*
*multiplication of these minute bodies (microbes), it is a consoling hope*
*that science will not always remain powerless before such enemies.*

- Louis Pasteur -

There is something quite addicting about providing medical care around the world in situations that are not always the safest. Most countries that need international assistance medically are developing nations with high rates of poverty and violence. The average U.S. citizen would not pick these locations for their next vacation, yet there is a calling for those who listen. The feeling of kissing my wife, sleeping in my own bed, having a warm shower, feeling clean, and eating real food is priceless upon returning from an expedition abroad. For the first few days I enjoy being home and readjust to the luxuries I possess. Soon after, however, I begin to feel it. It is like a vague hunger, not for food and water, but a hunger for adventure. The adventure calls for me like a lost lover. I hear her whispering my name as I try to ignore her. I try to move on with my responsibilities at home but her voice gets stronger. Over the course of a few weeks the voice overtakes me and I find myself on the computer scheduling my next trip.

What is it that draws me back, I wonder? The answer is not any one thing, but rather is a mix of altruism, sense of duty to society, and adventure. Much like Frodo setting off on his quest in *The Lord of the Rings* saga I did not seek out this mission, rather it sought me. After the earthquake, I knew I had to go and provide my services. The excitement and adventure became an addiction over time. I am the hero fighting my arch villain in Haiti: poverty. With this mentality I set off on my adventures to this Caribbean nation.

# The Michelle's

One day I met a wonderful family, the Michelle's. There was father, mother, and two children, Joseph and Rene Michelle. Rene was the older brother, aged six and role model for Joseph, the younger brother of four years of age. Joseph had always been fond of his older brother and albeit they were two years apart, they were like twins. Father had said that he could not separate the two. Wherever Rene went, Joseph had to follow and vice versa. They ate the same foods, had to wear the same clothes and play together. They were the best of friends and inseparable brothers. They lived in a tent city in the center of PaP, by the capitol building. Father and mother were doing well health wise but the children were sick. Through a translator, father began to tell me about their symptoms.

Rene had started with vomiting about four days prior. He had not been able to keep any of his food down and vomited up everything that was given to him, including water. The next day he began having loose stools which evolved over the next two days to a profuse watery diarrhea followed by a fever. His parents couldn't get Rene to the toilet fast enough and he soiled himself a few times. When Rene began having symptoms of vomiting and diarrhea, it was only a matter of time until Joseph followed suit. A couple of days later Joseph began with similar symptoms of wrenching abdominal pain followed by aggressive vomitus and diarrhea. The kids were not able to keep any food or water in their stomach and were progressively getting weaker. It was month 3 into the cholera epidemic and mother and father were slightly concerned that this may be cholera but were ashamed to seek medical help. In Haitian culture the thought amongst many was that cholera was a disease of the uneducated, lower class, those with poor hygiene, and those with misfortune. Thus, patients often wait until they are extremely sick before they seek medical care.

The Michelle family had waited a couple days before bringing their boys in for evaluation, hoping whatever it was would pass on its own. Both boys sat in our triage room outside the main ER. We had a policy of keeping suspected cholera out of the ER to prevent contamination. It was early in the morning and the boys were awake and active. First to catch my eyes was Rene. Rene's eyes were shallow, sunken in their sockets and his cheek bones high. His body had lost all its excess fluid and his bones were protruding. With each breath taken the small space between the ribs would expand visibly, clearly showcasing his bony anatomy. The knockoff brand spider man underwear he wore seemed a size to large, sagging off his bottom. He lay on his back in my gurney with his younger brother next to him, a carbon copy image. Both brothers were severely dehydrated and in need of urgent care or they would not make it through the night. We placed IVs in both kids and started rehydrating them with fluids. They were grumpy for about two minutes while the IV was being placed. As soon as the IV was secured and we let go of their arms, they forgot the whole trauma of having the needles poked in their arms and were back to giggling amongst one another. As resilient as children are, they continued to joke amongst one another whilst death lingered over their shoulders, unaware of the danger they were in.

As I stood next to the boys examining them we tried giving them some water to drink – which, turns out, was not a good idea. Joseph took a few sips and continued playing with his brother. As I examined him he turned his head to the side, looked me in the eyes, and vomited on my shoes. Having been doing this for a few days now, he was accustomed to vomiting and the next instant was back to giggling with Rene. The two of them lay together on the gurney like mirror images of each other. Each lay on his back with the left leg crossed across the right and the right arm resting on his head.

I stepped away to bleach my shoes, the only real way to kill the cholera bug. I returned and gave both kids a dose of anti-nausea medication along with an antibiotic to treat the cholera. Given the extremely high contractibility of this disease, hospitals in PaP learned not to manage cholera on their own. Instead, the government has set up designated cholera treatment centers where patients will receive appropriate medications and more importantly, rehydration. All we had to do was dial *300 from a mobile phone and the 'cholera police' would respond and transport patients to these centers. Our role was to stabilize and begin rehydration which we had accomplished. Stepping away and letting the boys relax and take in the new environment, we called *300 and soon enough a rusty old ambulance arrived our gates, ready to whisk the kids away to a cholera treatment center. While leaving, father said mêci and shook all of our hands on the way into the ambulance.

# Cholera in Haiti

Travelling to Haiti in 2011 I knew I would diagnose many cases of cholera. The cholera outbreak had been in full swing for a few months here in Haiti. For the most part, cholera is a disease that now affects developing countries with poor sanitation and hygiene techniques. Through education and clean running water we have virtually eradicated this foe from our homes in industrialized nations. Haiti had seen its fair share of cholera before but had mostly suppressed it for the past few decades. There were still occasional episodes of cholera usually imported from other countries, but nothing warranting major concern. In 2010, it was thought that the cholera bacterium was brought back to Haiti from foreign aid workers. Epidemiologic evidence suggests that it likely came with Sri Lankan workers who unknowingly passed the bacteria. Many people are silent carriers, which means they can harbor the bacteria without producing symptoms. These silent carriers acquired cholera in their home country and unwittingly brought the bug to Haiti, causing havoc.

Yearly, worldwide close to 5 million people are affected and in 2010 about 130,000 people are thought to have died from cholera around the world. Cholera reached Haiti in the fall of 2010 and from October through December of 2010 about 150,000 people contracted the disease and about 3,500 have died. The United Nations originally projected by the end of 2011 450,000 people would have been affected by cholera in Haiti. Now we are learning that this number is a gross underestimate. As of March 10th, 2011 252,640 people had been identified as having cholera and 4,672 have died, already surpassing the trend of the original estimate. The University of California at San Francisco estimates that by the end of 2011, close to 800,000 people will have been infected in Haiti alone and over 11,000 dead – that's a staggering 2-4% of the population of Haiti.

## Our Balrog: Cholera.

Remember the Balrog from *The Lord of the Rings* saga? The giant beast made of fire that Gandalf (then The Grey) warned the fellowship of. Balrog was the monster whose foe was no one and whose quest was that of only evil.

> Boromir: *What is this new devilry?*

> Gandalf: *A Balrog. A demon of the ancient world. This foe is beyond any of you. RUN!*

When I saw that scene it sent shivers down my spine. With hairs standing on edge and reflexes up I would watch Gandalf and the fellowship run from the Balrog to complete their mission.

> Gandalf: *You cannot pass! I am a servant of the Secret Fire, wielder of the Flame of Anor. The dark fire will not avail you, Flame of Udun! Go back to the shadow. You shall not pass!*

Culminating this harrowing escape was Gandalf facing off with the Balrog, only to fall down the abyss with his antithesis. Eventually Gandalf and the fellowship succeeded in their mission to save Middle-Earth.

How can watching such a primordial fictional character create such real intrigue? Maybe we genetically have a fear of ancient enemies, fictional or not. It makes sense, right? Our ancient predecessors millions of years ago learned quickly that pissing off a saber tooth tiger was a bad idea. Those who learned quickly to avoid them and taught their children this trait survived, those who didn't, well you can find them at the La Brea Tar Pits.

With time this trait was engrained in our genetics and passed on generation to generation. Millions of years later as I watch The Balrog threatening our fellowship on my couch and 52 inch LCD TV in surround sound, I still get the same "flight or fight" response my ancestors did – albeit a much more blunted response. With hairs on edge and eyes wide open I follow the vexing saga unfold. I know this is fiction I am watching but endocrine system does not. The endocrine system of the body is made up of numerous glands that secrete hormones which work throughout the body. One of those hormones is adrenaline, which causes the "flight or fight" response. Watching the drama unfold, my body can't tell the difference between movie and real life. Adrenaline flows and I am ready to fight or flight. This type of reaction to a perceived threat is one of our primordial instincts and we have learned, rightly so, to avoid the threat.

Many times we know our enemies when we see them and Balrog is easy enough to spot. But how about those that are not as easy? Those that need a microscope to find them? How does one recognize this threat let alone escape or avoid it?

# Drum roll please … {Enter Cholera}

Cholera is a pretty nasty disease. It causes uncontrollable diarrhea, abdominal pain, cramping, nausea, and vomiting. As the disease progresses the diarrhea gets worse and worse, eventually leading to dehydration. The diarrhea is characterized as 'rice-water' like in appearance. People have been known to lose upwards of 15 liters of water daily from diarrhea - that amounts to 7.5 two liter soda bottles. Clearly the human body cannot tolerate water loss like that for long. Along with losing water, we also lose essential salts in the diarrhea leading to electrolyte imbalances. Over the course of a few hours or days our kidneys shut down, then our brain and finally we die.

The bug that causes cholera is an ancient foe – a bacterium called *Vibrio cholera*. Having been around for millions of years it has claimed millions if not billions of lives. It is spread by poor hygiene – fecal contents contaminating our drinking water/food, etc. The bacterium swims its way to the small intestine and sets up camp. From there it begins to multiply and starts producing a toxin which causes the severe diarrhea. We learned quickly that even if we cannot see our foe, drinking water downstream from camp was a bad idea. Children are particularly susceptible as are the elderly. Interestingly, through research we know that people with O type blood are more susceptible than other blood groups. On the contrary, the gene for cystic fibrosis protects against infection. Those who have the gene for cystic fibrosis but do not have the disease have an advantage at resisting cholera.

When identified and treated early, cholera is fairly manageable. The mainstay of treatment is fluid rehydration and antibiotics. With time, rehydration, and patience most people recover. Many, however, do not seek care until their cholera is severe at which time it may be too late to prevent organ damage and death.

The Michelle children fortunately sought medical care in a timely fashion and will survive their brush with cholera. The same cannot be said for the thousands and millions who have lost their lives to this vicious Balrog – an ancient foe that we will continue to fight with modern medicine in our quest to save mankind.

The Michelle brothers resilience helped keep the mood up throughout this dire situation. It is amazing how kids tend to bounce back from serious illness or injury. Kids have it right – they don't spend hours and days groping or crying about a situation. Instead, they move on and continue doing what they do best, being happy. I try to keep that happy child-like outlook on life as much as possible. In a way, it's how I can let things like death bounce right off me and how I stay sane in such depressing situations. Months later, when I held the hand of one of my close patients who was dying at home from liver cancer, I told him the story of Rene and Joseph. We both laughed and agreed that the world would be a better place if we could look at life as kids do. After he died, remembering those boys laying on the gurney giggling after having an IV put in kept me from crying that night as I coped with his death. I prayed they survived their bout with cholera, but knew either way their childhood spirit would never die.

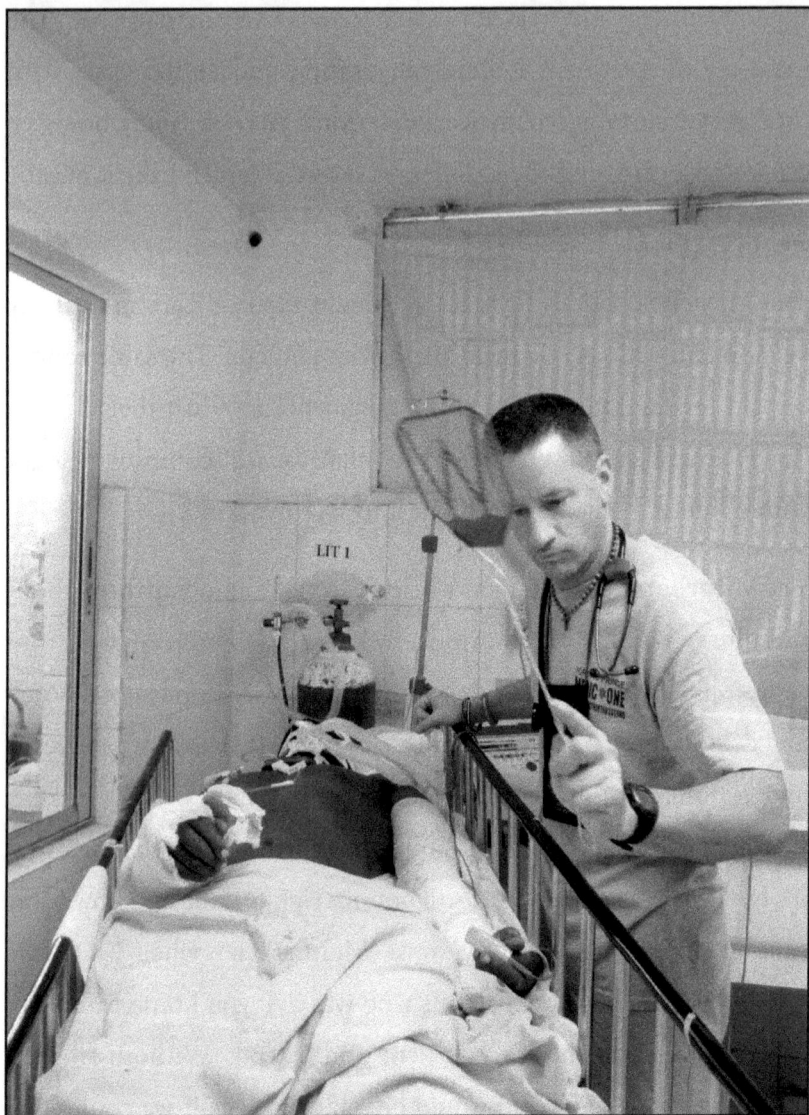

Critical Care Nurse swatting away mosquitoes and flies from a patient in the ICU

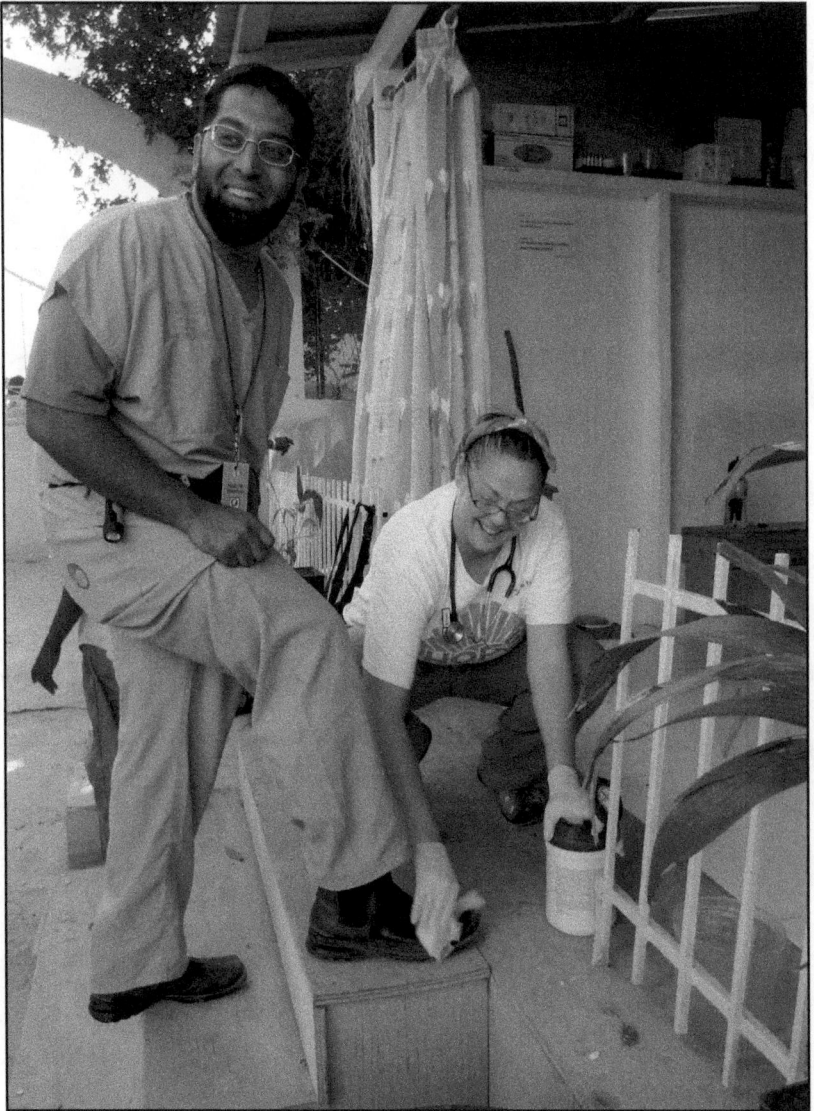
Decontaminating from cholera after Joseph vomited on my shoes.

# Night Sweats

*While the Bush administration is prepared to spend $100 billion to rid Iraq of WMD, it has been unwilling to spend more than 0.2% of that sum... this year on the Global Fund to Fight AIDS, Tuberculosis and Malaria.*

- Jeffrey Sachs -

Have you ever had night sweats, true night sweats? Waking up in the middle of the night with your sheets soaked through, needing to be changed? For most of us, it usually lasts a day or so and is associated with having a "cold." When it continues on for longer periods of time, it can be scary. The differential diagnosis of night sweats is quite broad, including fever, stress, anxiety, infection, and cancer. In Haiti, however, night sweats are one of a handful of things until proven otherwise: malaria, tuberculosis, dengue fever, typhoid, or HIV. The last, of course, is easily identifiable by blood testing. The others, however, are a bit wilier and can masquerade as other conditions making the critical time from symptom onset to diagnosis longer than it should be and blunting the ability to cure and treat the disease in a timely fashion. Imagine having to go weeks on weeks with unremitting night sweats – miserable to say the least.

## Mr. Jamiel

Mr. Jamiel was a twenty-two-year-old brought in by his family complaining of weakness, confusion, and fevers. For the past three days or so, he had fevers and chills along with a general feeling of malaise. He had been noticing night sweats for the past six weeks but thought nothing of it. He would soak his sheets through and through. There was such a stench of sweat that every two days he was washing his sheets.

The fevers are what bothered him the most. The fever was worse when he would wake up in the morning but would often persist throughout the day. He had also been complaining of headache and nausea with vomiting for the past few days. No one else at home was sick, so he could not pinpoint where he got this sickness. Over the past few days his mother said he started acting confused and forgetting things. This morning she found him in bed lethargic and very hard to arouse. When he did open his eyes, he mumbled words that no one could make out. She knew something was wrong and urgently brought him to our hospital.

When Mr. Jamiel arrived in our tent hospital, he was confused and lethargic. He was a good looking young man, tall and skinny but looked like he had just come back from war. His Nike shirt was torn and worn out. His jeans were holey with brown fecal stains on the back. There was a stench of urine permeating the atmosphere around him, as if he had not been cleaned in a few days. He would open his eyes to pain but otherwise was unresponsive. His temperature was 102 degrees Fahrenheit. IV fluids were started and basic labs sent.

In malaria endemic regions fever is always a tip off for malaria. Most of the time malaria itself does not lend to nausea and vomiting. In severe cases though, it can sometimes spread to the brain and cause vague symptoms like headache and nausea – this is called cerebral malaria. On exam, he was severely dehydrated. It was obvious he hadn't been eating or drinking for a few days. A couple hours later the malaria test from his blood came back positive, confirming my clinical diagnosis. Since he was clinically dehydrated and confused, he was admitted for intravenous IV fluids, anti-malarial medications, and observation. Jamiel was very sick and his condition was fragile at best.

# Malaria

Malaria is caused by a small parasite called *Plasmodium*. This parasite is carried from person to person by a vector (carrier agent). The vectors are the female (males don't feed on humans) *Anopheles* mosquito. Once infected, malaria causes fevers, chills, shaking, and an overall feeling of lethargy. This may lead to headache, nausea, and stomach pain. The classic presentation of malaria is cyclical fevers; that is, fevers that come and go usually at night or in the morning. When the fevers come, people generally feel lethargic and sick. Once the fever subsides, they tend to feel a bit better and go on with their everyday lives. As the disease progresses, patients may describe joint, neck, and back pains. In severe cases the parasite can infect the brain and cause confusion, coma, and ultimately death.

Malaria is a worldwide problem and The World Health Organization (WHO) estimates that it causes over 200 million cases of fever every year. In 2010 over 600,000 people died from Malaria. For the most part, malaria spreading mosquitoes tend to hover around the equatorial region given the humidity and rain fall. Thus, malaria is seen equally throughout the world in these areas. Treatment for malaria in Haiti (a malaria endemic region) is fairly simple – a medication called chloroquine. Through time and with the excess usage of chloroquine many parts of the world have *Plasmodium* species that have developed resistance to chloroquine. With resistant cases more expensive and dangerous drugs have to be used. Luckily, Haitian malaria is still chloroquine sensitive.

Treating malaria in Haiti is rather easy since chloroquine is an old, inexpensive, and readily available medication. When patients complain of fever with no other obvious source of the fever (a cold or other infection), malaria is high on the list of causative agents. Presumptively treating with chloroquine is never the wrong thing to do. At the time, the only medication we had in our hospital was chloroquine which we began giving Mr. Jamiel.

Through my interpreter, I was able to better understand Mr. Jamiel's story. He and his family of six were displaced by the earthquake and were staying in one of the numerous tent cities that had sprung up to house the two million homeless. Prior to the earthquake they lived in a concrete home about six hundred square feet. Now they were confined to a tent. What was originally a three-person tent was now accommodating seven. His family recalled that three days ago he was his normal self but had been complaining of chills and mild fever. Later that day, he began having a severe fever. I asked how high the fever was – a silly question to ask. Some families do not even have toilet paper; where would they get a thermometer from? Remembering where I was, I continued with the history.

All night he maintained a high fever and was shaking in bed. His sheets were soaked in sweat. He awoke the next morning with a severe headache. It was the worst headache of his life – crushing, diffuse, and the pain made him nauseous. As the day went on he began acting more and more confused. His family was concerned when he became disoriented. He didn't know where he was and

114

responded to the family's questioning with gibberish no one could understand.

As the hours went on he became more and more somnolent. Later that night, he was unresponsive and the family decided to bring him to the hospital. Lab tests confirmed that he had malaria. His clinical status suggested it had spread to the brain. In the United States when there is concern for a brain infection we perform a spinal tap to look at the fluid to determine the causative agent and the medications that are needed. With the limited resources at the time, a spinal tap was out of the question. We treated patients mostly on our clinical judgment.

Jamiel was receiving anti-malarial medications and copious IV fluids. He was sweating so profusely that he required close to 6 liters of fluids daily. After a few hours we were able to obtain a stronger malaria medication used for suspected cases of cerebral malaria. We began giving him this medication hoping that it would help him turn the corner and recover. Due to the dire conditions and lack of resources we had no IV poles to hang the fluid bags on. Instead, a small twine was tied to each end of the tent. When an IV bag was in use, a small hook was placed on that twine to elevate the bag. IV fluids are crucial in treating many diseases as they contain electrolytes and water essential in keeping the body hydrated and in enabling the immune system to fight off infection. Even with the appropriate treatment regimen for malaria, Jamiel's condition did not seem to be improving. He continued to have drenching sweats and fevers overnight.

The next day I reviewed his chart to ensure he was receiving the appropriate medications and quantities of fluids. The odds were against him – cerebral malaria carries a grim prognosis. He had a fever of 102 degrees Fahrenheit and his blood pressure was unstable. When people become septic (meaning an infection spreads to the blood and organs), they often cannot maintain an adequate blood pressure. Inflammatory markers released by the immune system combined with toxins from the invading parasite cause the blood vessels to dilate. Dilation (widening) of the blood vessels leads to a drop in blood pressure. When the blood pressure drops vital organs such as the kidneys, heart, and brain do not get enough blood to work properly and slowly die.

A normal person's blood pressure should be around 120/80 mmHg. Jamiel's blood pressure was 60/40 mmHg, and his skin was cold, clammy, and pale. At this point, medications and IV fluids were about all we could do. Time and fate would determine his outcome. I met with his family and urged them to pray for him.

Over the next few hours, I kept a close eye on his progress. He continued to lose about one to two liters of water from sweating. We ran the IV fluids as fast as we could just to catch up with the fluid lost from sweating. His blood pressure was not improving, and thus far he had received over fifteen liters of fluids – an astounding amount when one recalls that the human body has about five liters of blood. He was mostly lethargic but when he did wake, he would gaze about as if staring past his family members standing in front of him. A few incoherent words would be mumbled and just like that he would drift back into his state of sleep. Night came and he was still fighting. Blood pressure was low but held stable. He was still febrile but alive. We kept giving him medications and fluids and rode the storm through the night.

Early the next morning I did my rounds. The first patient I evaluated was Jamiel. His temperature read 103.9 Fahrenheit. When I looked back at his vital signs overnight the trend was clear and it did not look good. Going on three documented days now he had fevers over 102 degrees Fahrenheit, blood pressures in the septic range, and a heart rate over 100. A normal resting heart rate should be well below 100 beats per minute, likely around 70 or so. His heart rate of 120 was akin to what I would expect mine to be if I was walking on the treadmill. He had maintained a rate like this for at least three days now, practically using up all his fluids and muscle storage in this constant state of stress. He was burning out.

Later that day, now the third day of his admission, I noticed his breathing was becoming more and more shallow. He was not responding to pain and not opening his eyes. As death nears, our breathing pattern changes: we take smaller, shallower breaths. At this point, I knew he was heading down a one-way road from which he could not return. I spent some time explain the grave situation to the family. I expected them to react as my patients' families in the United States often did: frustrated, angry, tired, sad – overall emotional. Ironically they simply nodded their heads in understanding and continued on with their prayers. With all the death from devastation thrown at them unexpectedly throughout their lives in Haiti, it seemed a gradual death from a known killer was a bit more tolerable.

The family continued to pray and I continued to provide medical treatment. Later that day, around 4 in the afternoon, Mr. Jamiel's heart went into a terminal rhythm. The build of toxins in the blood and stress on the body was too much for his heart to bear. The cells in his heart were damaged and couldn't perform their duties. After a few minutes of an abnormal heart rhythm his heart finally began to slow. 180 beats per minute – 160 – 120 – 100 – 80 – 70 – 50 – 40 – 40 – 40 – 30 – 30 – 20 – 0. Mr. Jamiel peacefully passed and his family wept quietly at his bedside.

In medicine we are trained to deal with death and dying. Over time we become accustomed to it and, for a lack of better words, become desensitized to some extent. We still empathize with those grieving of course, but we have to separate our emotions from the recurrent death. It is a fine line we walk: providing medical care while avoiding deep emotional attachment. It is nearly impossible to avoid some level of emotional bondage with our patients. When they pass, it hurts. With time we learn to "medicalize", as I like to say, our patients. Instead of referring to Mr. Jamiel as such, we call him "the malaria" or others as "the foot infection", "the diabetic", or (my personal favorite) "the vag bleeder." In a way this dehumanizes the case by removing the one thing all humans have in common yet makes us unique – a name.

After all, doctors are just regular people. We cry when our friends die and we bleed when we are cut as well. Having to say good bye to a

*Night Sweats*

patient I've cared for, often times for years, as they die in their home or the hospital is never easy. Remove the name from the patient and we're left treating not John Allen, but "the foot." It's a lot easier on us when "the foot" dies instead of John Allen. By doing so we ensure our own sanity in being able to let go and move on to the next battle.

As Mr. Jamiel's family wept, I felt my heart sink but immediately pulled it back up and moved on to my next patient. An anonymous quote I read a while back came to mind, summarized:

*Death is not a physician's enemy.*

*He is our long lost brother to whom we will reunite.*

*It is never a failure to accept him,*

*Only, to deny him*

*What is rightfully his.*

## The Superbug

Over the years there have been numerous news stories featuring the "superbug," a microbe that has developed resistance to the medications we usually utilize in its treatment. Most recent in the news have been stories about MRSA (methicillin-resistant *Staphylococcus aureus*) and the severe gangrenous skin infections it can cause. *Staphylococcus aureus* is a bacterium that is part of our normal skin flora and fauna, causing no problem for the majority of us. In certain immunosuppressed individuals such as diabetics, the flora of our skin can overgrow its territory causing an infection that needs to be treated. Classically, the treatment for staph infections was a penicillin family medication. With time resistance to this family of medications developed, hence the evolution of MRSA which requires different antibiotics for treatment.

The inherent difficulty with treating any bacteria or virus is the worry about drug resistance. Darwin's law of natural selection and survival of the fittest fundamentally comes to fruition on the microbial level. Humans take nine months to replicate, whereas microbe replication rates are measured in minutes to hours. Evolutionary changes are usually described as happening over generations. Over tens or hundreds of generations genes and traits slowly change.

Take for example the classic case of the peppered moths, taught in biology courses around the world. In England the predominant color of peppered moths was a light-colored hue, which allowed them to camouflage on the naturally light-colored tree bark. Their natural predators were birds and the camouflage protected the moths. During the industrial revolution in the 1800s pollution and soot deposition began to occur in the forests, changing the trees' light hue to a darker color. The change in the color of the trees disrupted the camouflage of the moths and they began to die as they were now visible to their predators. As they were hunted, moths of different colors began having an evolutionary advantage. Previously the darker moths would have been the easy prey, yet because of the darker soot-covered trees these moths began surviving as they were better camouflaged. Over time their numbers grew as they mated and replicated. Slowly the color of their progeny changed. Soon enough the moth population was no longer light colored but rather evolved to take on a darker tone overall, thus ensuring survival of the species as a whole. That was evolution.

Evolutionary changes, which take hundreds or thousands of years in large animals, take merely months or years in fast-replicating life forms. Microbes are the fastest replicators on earth and can incorporate evolutionary changes in their genetic material rapidly. With repeated exposure to medications and incomplete antibiotic courses, microbes that survive the antimicrobial medications become "superbugs," resistant to our alchemy. Through time these bugs then replicate and evolve like the moths of England. With microbes, this evolutionary change may only take a few years or months. This rapid change proves to be quite the hindrance to modern pharmacological treatment. The next time you are given a course of antibiotics, make sure to complete the course as instructed even if you are feeling better, lest your co-existing and pathogenic bacteria will develop resistance as well.

## Tuberculosis

Small donated tents, commonly called 'shelter in a box,' were distributed to displaced victims shortly after the earthquake. Originally meant for temporary housing only, most of these tents became permanent residences for families. These tents often ended up on the 'tent black market' and would be sold for around $50 USD for a small two-person tent to $200 USD for a larger five-person tent. In Haitian terms $200 USD could feed a family of five for three months – a significant amount of money.

In the field hospital we used these tents as isolation wards, kept away from the larger general ward tents. The first tent was the morgue, where bodies were placed until they could be picked up. The other two tents were isolation tents where patients with severely communicable diseases such as tuberculosis (TB) were admitted.

Tuberculosis is a disease caused by the bacteria *Mycobacterium tuberculosis*, which can affect multiple organs in the body. Classically we think of TB affecting the lungs predominately, but it can also affect the abdomen, brain, urinary tract, and even the skin. It is often a slow-growing disease that is endemic in developing countries. Pulmonary TB (infection in the lung) is the most common manifestation of TB and is something that develops over years in most people. It is primarily spread by cough, but can also be spread by saliva. Not everyone who is exposed to TB actually contracts the disease. Most are able to mount an immune response and prevent TB from infecting their cells. In others, TB just stays in the body asleep for years (what we call latent TB) until something wakes it up and it becomes active TB. At the highest risk of acquiring TB are people whose immune system cannot fight off an exposure such as diabetics, patients with cancer or HIV, and those with other immunosuppressant diseases.

Pulmonary TB is a slowly progressing disease process. Classically a patient will often go for months or years without knowing they have TB until it causes significant symptoms. Eventually they will present with weight loss, fevers, chills, night sweats, cough with brown-tinged rusty-colored sputum, or frank blood in their sputum. By that point the TB is no longer latent and has converted over to an active infection of the lungs. The weight loss is often significant with patients losing anywhere from 10-30% of their body weight. The combination of weight loss and the infection from the TB keeps the immune system so busy that it cannot fight off other dangerous bugs. For example, the bacterium that in healthy individuals causes mild symptoms such as sniffles may cause a severe lung infection such as pneumonia in TB patients. This in turn leads to breathing difficulty and scarred lung tissue which eventually causes respiratory failure and death. TB claims about two million lives yearly worldwide the majority of which are in developing nations. When identified early enough and without other co-morbid conditions, TB is usually treatable. In the United States physicians perform a routine TB tests by injecting a bit of reactant in the skin and inspecting the patient's skin response in three days. If the TB test is positive we send the patient for a chest X-ray. If nothing shows up on the X-ray they are considered X-ray negative. Chest X-ray negative patients are given the diagnosis of latent TB and are offered six to nine months of medication to prevent TB activation. Patients with findings on the X-ray consistent with TB are called X-ray positive patients. X-ray positive patients have active TB that needs multiple medications (often three) for six to twelve months. Multiple medications are used in active TB to prevent resistance by ensuring the bug is killed by hitting hard and fast, so to speak. Patients with TB are usually treated quite easily as an outpatient if the disease is identified early enough – which is sadly not always the case.

# Robert

Robert was a young sixteen-year-old previously healthy male with no medical problems. He came to our hospital extremely short of breath to the point he needed to be placed on oxygen continuously just to be able to speak to us. Instead of enjoying his youth by playing soccer or being out with friends, he had been confined to his home for the past three months. What started off as a cough had turned into something much worse - TB.

Per his mother about four months ago he started having an intermittent raspy cough which seemed to come and go. Over time the cough progressed to a chronic daily cough and he began having blood-tinged sputum. About the second month in he started having profuse night sweats. He described waking up in the morning and feeling as if he had just taken a shower – his clothes were drenched in sweat. His weight began to drop and with it his energy level and interest in what he once enjoyed. About ten weeks into his symptoms he was finally diagnosed as having TB by a doctor at the local general hospital, which was a government hospital in downtown PaP.

An appropriate three-drug regimen was started after diagnosis. His mother was responsible for his care and confirmed that she provided him every dose, having missed maybe only one or two doses throughout his course at most. About six weeks into treatment he was not doing any better. He continued to lose weight and have bloody sputum. He was taken to the general hospital where his drug regimen was changed in the hopes of fighting the infection better.

124

Robert's energy level continued to plummet and finally, he was unable to care for himself. His mother could not get him out of bed to use the restroom or take a shower. She tried feeding him but he would not eat; he would just say, "I'm too tired." Slowly his respiratory rate began to increase and he found himself short of breath to the point that he could not finish sentences when he was speaking. At that point his mother brought him in to our field hospital for evaluation.

Most cases of TB tend to respond fairly well with the multidrug regimen over the course of six to nine months. However, there are cases that do not respond to the standard treatment and develop resistance to our routine modality. These strains of TB develop multidrug resistance and are extremely difficult to treat. This TB superbug is referred to as MDR TB (multidrug resistant Tuberculosis).

When Robert's story was recounted it was clear that he had developed MDR TB. For some time now he was given all the medications as prescribed yet his TB bug was not responding to treatment. When he arrived at the hospital his breathing was labored, rapid, and shallow. A chest X-ray showed diffuse lung disease and his oxygen saturation in the blood was measured at 89 percent (normal around 97 percent or higher). I provided him with our standard concoction of TB medications, antibiotics to fight off any secondary lung infections, oxygen, and IV fluids. We didn't have the special TB meds he was on as those were quite difficult to acquire. He had to be started on a generic TB medication regimen. Since he had confirmed TB he was placed in an isolation tent outside the main tent area. Once or twice a day the nurses and I would go out to check up on him. When his oxygen tank would run out he would call ancillary staff to replace it. This would often take an hour to get done and he would go for a significant amount of time with no supplemental oxygen. Things tend to run at their own pace in Haiti and urgency is not a universal concept. His mother, who was with him throughout the stay, slept with him and against our advice never wore a mask.

I had to watch poor Robert slowly succumb to his infection. The TB superbug had infected his lungs so badly that he would nearly faint when taken off the oxygen. Over the course of the next day he continued to struggle for life. His oxygen level never went over 90 percent on supplemental oxygen and his mental status was waning. He would sometimes know where he was and acknowledge his mother and at other times be lethargic and mute. I knew he did not have more than a few hours of life at worst and a few days at best. Either way he would die without the proper medications; that much was certain.

Unfortunately the TB medications we had were the standard first-line regimen, which he had been on and developed resistance to already. The medications he needed were expensive and hard to find. I called numerous hospitals/pharmacies/aid organizations in the area and none had the medications. Finally Partners in Health's award-winning TB treatment center in Cange had the facility to manage this case. They told me to send him to Cange, a three-hour drive from PaP, and they would be happy to take care of him. At their facility they would be able to isolate the TB bug and figure out what medications it was sensitive to and tailor a specific treatment for him; seemed simple enough except for the fact that he was dying *now* and would not make a three-hour car ride. Had he presented to our clinic even one day sooner, his outcome might be different.

We are often asked how long a patient is going to live. This is the ultimate question we all avoid answering. Every patient is different and their response to an illness even more so. Thus there is no magical equation or calculator to know when someone will die. We make educated guesses based on some science but mostly anecdotal experiences. Even though Robert's chance of surviving the car ride was slim, I knew he did have a chance of making it. We worked feverishly that night to arrange a car, driver, and oxygen tanks to take him on the journey in the morning. I informed his mother of this plan to which she was agreeable. I also discussed the idea of intubating Robert by placing a tube in his throat to help him breathe. If we secured his airway by having a tube, we could ensure he was breathing the whole ride over by providing oxygen and breathing for him with a bag. Robert and his mother both refused this – they did not want to have a tube put down his throat even if it was only done as a preventative measure to avoid catastrophe during the transport. We never try to transport unstable patients because bad things tend to always happen in the worst situations, such as a 3 hour car ride to another hospital. Still, Robert and his mother were both adamantly refusing intubation. We went to bed not knowing what the morning would bring but hoping for the sun to rise on another day of life and new hopes for Robert.

The next day I checked on Robert and knew this was going to be a difficult journey. He was drenched in sweat, awake, and with a raspy voice asked if he was ready to leave. I informed him he would leave as soon as he received his morning medications and fluids. Looking at his chart, I noted that his temperature was 101 degrees Fahrenheit. When I checked his blood oxygen level it was 82 percent even on maximum supplementary oxygen. I asked again if they would allow me to intubate him prior to his departure for his safety. Once again they declined. About an hour later he was ready to go and was loaded into the vehicle along with a couple of oxygen tanks and one of our nurses to ensure the oxygen kept running. The mother said her prayers and I said mine – and with that they were off.

I continued with my duties for the day and about two hours later received a phone call from my nurse. An hour after embarking Robert's breathing became shallower and labored. The oxygen was at maximum flow and he was tiring out. He began showing signs of respiratory fatigue such as nasal flaring (opening up the nostrils widely to take in as much air as possible, much like what we do when we are exercising) and using his abdominal muscles to breathe. He was tiring out and his body had no energy to continue the exhaustive process of living. The nurse gave him some morphine to slow down his breathing hoping that would help him absorb more oxygen. She increased his IV fluids. The nurse did all she could but he finally took his last breath of air and expired. The TB had won. The vehicle turned around and was on its way back. I felt beat. I had tried everything I could including arranging transport to a more equipped facility, yet in the end, I had been defeated. Frustration began to set in as this was the second patient in less than two days who had died

128

under my watch. If only I could have intubated him before he left, he probably would have made the trip. I felt like I had failed.

When the party returned I gave my condolences to the mother, who was sobbing. Prior to coming to us she had the idea that her son might die, but arranging the transport and the hustle of getting him ready to go gave her hope – gave me hope. I did not know what to tell her and simply put my hand around her and let her cry on my shoulder. After about ten minutes of grieving she was done. She thanked me for my time and said she had to go back home to take care of her other children and husband. On her way out she said in Creole, "Unfortunately, I may still need that ride to Cange." "Why?" I asked. She responded, "My other son has been coughing for two weeks now." And so the vicious cycle of life and death continued for her family and for Haiti, and their battle with TB was just beginning.

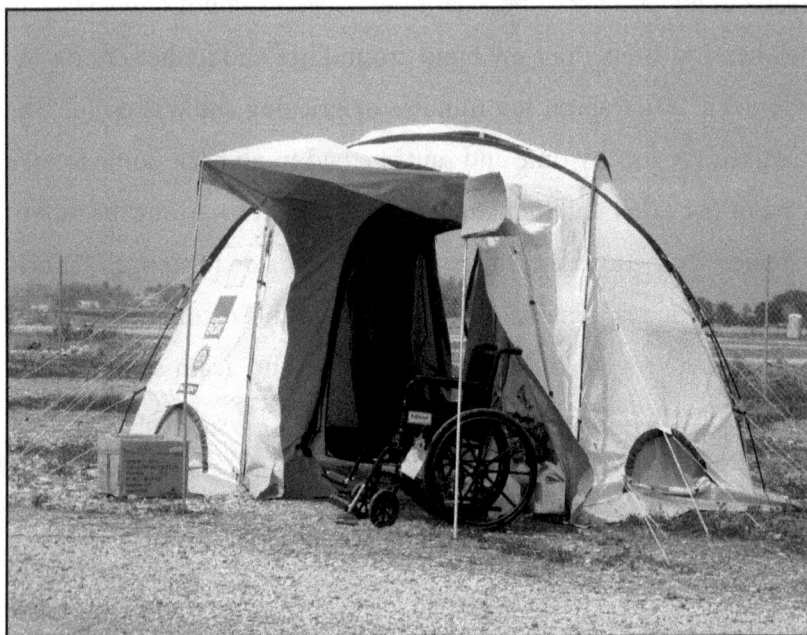

TB isolation tent

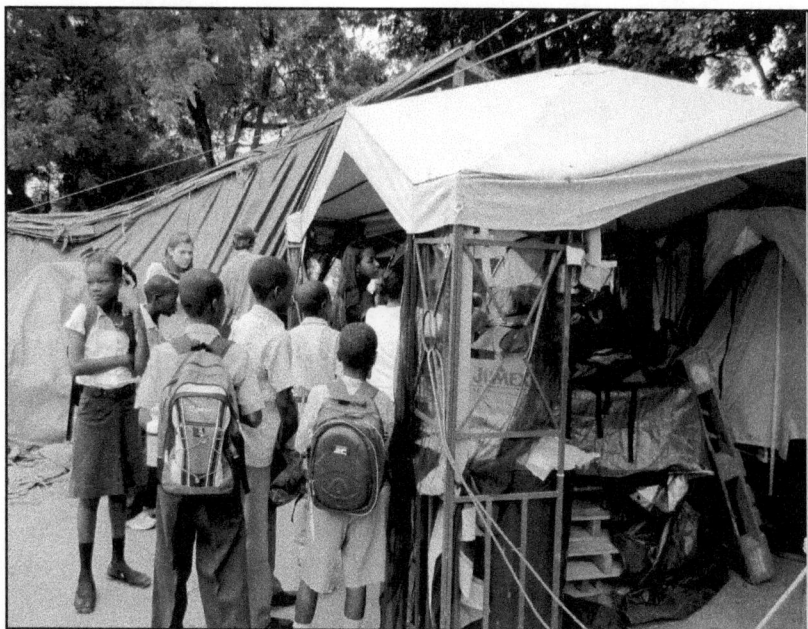
Children being treated at one of the many Dominican Republic
tent clinics.

# Dance of the Mind

*There are people in the world so hungry, that God cannot appear to them except in the form of bread.*

- Mahatma Gandhi -

It was early in the afternoon when my phone rang. Many calls come and go through the hospital mobile phone I carried and I expected nothing unusual with this one - expecting someone from another hospital needing a CT scan, or medication, or possibly transfer of care. I answered the phone "Hello, Bernard Mevs Hospital" as I always do in English. This helps the speaker on the other side know that I speak English and if they do not, then they state so at the onset. This time the caller responded in English with a Franco accent and began to tell me about Pauline.

Calling another hospital in Haiti and asking to transfer someone there is a hard fought battle. All of the NGO's that have hospitals are strapped for resources and are doing the best with what little they have. Even so, we know some hospitals have certain facilities that others do not and often try to barter transfers. Nine times out of ten the transfer is in to our hospital rather than out. We have the best acute care facilities of the NGO hospitals including ventilators, operating rooms, imaging (including a full CT scanner and 3D x-rays), laboratory, and knowledgeable and accessible staff. While on the phone my colleague and I both knew he would really have to sell this case for me to accept the transfer since we were short staffed during the New Year holidays (and thus accepted fewer patients).

Pauline was an eight year old child brought to MSF Belgium's Hospital in status epilepticus. Status epilepticus is a condition whereby the brain has a seizure that just won't stop - a sort of marathon of seizures if you will. She was found by her parents the day before having a seizure in her bedroom. Her parents took her to a medicine man for herbal treatment. The medicine man told her parents Pauline was 'dancing in her mind' and need remedies to wake her up. When this did not help, a good eighteen hours later, her parents brought her to MSF Belgium. Dr. Franco told me they had tried numerous doses of anti-seizure medications to no avail. Pauline kept seizing.

For most adults, status eplipeticus for such a long period of time has a very poor prognosis. While the body is seizing the brain doesn't get the oxygen it needs to survive and brain damage is a major concern. We try to stabilize status epilepticus in minutes - Pauline had been seizing for almost 24 hours now. Children, however, are resilient and bounce back from what many adults would die from. Given she was a child, I knew Pauline deserved a fighting chance as she still had some hope of recovery. Had the call been about an adult patient, I likely would have declined the transfer given the poor likelihood of survival and our limited resources. Triaging is a sad truth in Haiti. With the paucity of resources we have to use our clinical judgment in deciding which patients have the highest chance of survival before accepting them and using up one of our precious beds. Pauline's transfer I accepted. She would arrive in about 30 - 45 minutes and I had a lot to do to get ready for her in the meantime.

Today I had a local Haitian physician, Dr. Rimelle, training in the ER. In Haiti a residency, or post medical school training, is not required to practice medicine. Most physicians choose what type of medicine they would like to practice and often shadow another physician for some time before setting up their own shop. Dr. Rimelle decided she wanted to be a general pediatrician. It being

Haiti of course, even pediatricians see adults. She would still see patients of all ages but chose to focus on children. Dr. Rimelle would work a few shifts in the ER on her own during the week and when we were working together we would find procedures and other teaching opportunities. I told her about Pauline and that she would need to be intubated upon arrival. As I had hoped, Dr. Rimelle asked if she could do the intubation under my supervision. We came up with a delegation of duties and I informed my team of the transfer and we all readied for her arrival. Our pharmacist drew up pediatric doses of anti-seizure medications, nurses got their supplies ready, I prepared our intubation tray - and with that we were ready for Pauline.

About an hour after preparations were made, the MSF ambulance arrived. In pulled an old Landcruiser. The 1990's white Toyota Landcruiser is an iconic international vehicle seen all over the world. It is what a true SUV should be. Built solidly, the vehicle has a "don't mess with me" kind of attitude; ready to take on any terrain including water with the built in snorkel providing air to the engine for combustion even when partially submerged. When I was younger my dream vehicle was the 1960 FJ-40 Toyota Landcruiser. In 1951 the Landcruiser was the first vehicle to climb to the top of Mount Fuji and the highest climb of any vehicle up until then. It was the Japanese Imperial Army's response to the ever popular British Land Rover and the American Jeep. Since its production, the Landcruiser has evolved drastically covering all terrains from the Australian outback (considered by many off-road enthusiasts as being one of the most trying in the world and where many off road vehicles are tested) to the urban sprawl – making it the longest running production line vehicle in Toyota's impressive history.

In the late 1980's, early 1990's Toyota released the Landcruiser series 80. During this time many units were produced for police, military, wildlife, and patrol uses. As they were used and replaced with newer models, the series 80 vehicles were sold in bulk to developing nations, NGOs, and other organizations on a budget. The series 80 Landcruisers were particularly desirable as there were millions sold throughout the years making maintenance and parts fairly easy to come by. Many NGOs in Haiti had bought these vehicles and removed the back seats to convert the Landcruiser into a makeshift ambulance.

As the series 80 Landcruiser made its way through our gates I immediately noticed the MSF emblem on the hood and the standard MSF 'no weapons allowed' insignia on the windows. I always found it inspiring that the organization MSF was categorically opposed to firearms regardless of the use or user in its vehicles. MSF had a universal policy that maintained a neutral weapons free environment in all its vehicles, making it a benign entity in an otherwise dangerous environment. Sirens and lights blaring, the Toyota pulled past our green front gates into our driveway. The driver was a Haitian who waived at me as he drove past and stopped where I instructed. Inside I could see two Haitian passengers on either side of a gurney and a Caucasian gentleman beside them. I opened the back gate and a tall, slender man with strikingly European features jumped out of the vehicle with an urgency rarely seen in Haiti. Shaking his hand I saw the deep wrinkles around his eyes we all tend to get when working in

*Dance Of The Mind*

Haiti from lack of sleep. He saluted me with "Bonjour" followed by "Hello I am Doctor Anid …" in a heavy French accent that reminded me of Jean-Claude Van Damme.

As the doors swung open I saw an older Haitian couple sitting on either side of a stretcher laid in the middle of the truck. Dr. Anid introduced the parents, whom up until now I thought must have been the grandparents of this child given their age. They were considerably older than what I would have expected for parents of an eight year old. Father was wearing an old red plaid long sleeve shirt on top of worn out denim jeans. He looked to be in his sixties; weathered skin, wrinkled eyes, and weighed no more than 115 pounds. Mother sat across from him and wore a simple blue dress with dirt and sweat stains throughout. Her hair was in tight corn rolls. She looked as if she had not slept for a few days.

Between both parents lay Pauline. Dr. Anid told me she was eight but she looked no older than six. Poverty and malnutrition tend to make children grow slower and Pauline's growth was obviously subpar. She too had on a simple blue dress, a school uniform, but hers was stained with all sorts of bodily fluids – blood around the arms with a single IV line in one hand, vomitus over most of the chest, fecal matter and urine staining the lower half. Beads of sweat ran down her forehead and a stench of bodily fluids permeated the air. I imagined the smell akin to sweaty gym clothes dunked in urine and feces and run through the dryer.

Ron, a Haitian once told me "We don't have many clothes here in Haiti, but the clothes we do have we work hard to take care of. I never let myself or any of my family members walk out of the house with any stains on our clothes…it's our culture." Remembering this cultural standard, I looked down at Pauline covered in excrement and her parents on either side wearing tattered and dirty clothes. Mother and Father's clothes, however, were not only stained but showed evidence of having been weathered. These outfits were likely one of the better ones the family possessed yet were blatantly old and worn, beyond repair in some places. It was obvious at that point that this family was the poorest of Haiti.

I looked back down at Pauline and saw that she was shaking her entire body, as if in a silent dance, lost in her own mind. Her eyes were open yet not looking at anything. Her seizures were subtle but ongoing. Through her half open dress her chest was visible. As malnourished as she was I could count each and every one of her ribs – she looked like the anatomy drawings we all studied during medical school. A picture from *Netter's Atlas of Anatomy* came to mind (the timeless anatomy text nearly all medical students in the U.S. and other countries used during their training). Ironically, poverty had perfectly outlined each of her immaculate features.

We moved Pauline on to our gurney and rushed her in to our ER.

---

Pauline was in our ER and nurses started finding a vein to place a second IV line for good vascular access. In times of emergencies we try to have at least two working IV lines. This allows us to run fluids through one and meds through another. EMTs were cutting off her clothes to allow for an unobstructed and thorough secondary survey and evaluation for injury. Another nurse was attaching electrocardiography (ECG) leads to check the rhythms of the heart. Medical students started their physical exam by listening to her heart and lungs. Translators were talking to the family obtaining more of her history as we worked. In the organized chaos that ensued there were always 8-10 people surrounding Pauline at any given time, each with a specific role. As the team leader I strategically placed myself at the head of the bed with Dr. Rimelle shouting out orders. Like a well-practiced orchestra, I conducted my team with finesse. We were ready for this. Watch any individual and it seemed like a slow task but sit back and observe the whole team work in unison and the concerto was coming together. Within 5 minutes we had good venous access with two IV lines in place, heart monitors on, a basic evaluation done, and were ready to secure her airway.

I asked for anti-seizure and paralyzing medications to be given. Our clinical pharmacist had the doses ready and a nurse pushed both. A few seconds later Pauline's shaking began to slow and finally cease. Her dance had been stopped by our medications. She was no longer seizing and her breathing had stopped – the desired effect we had induced, a sort of temporary death. By paralyzing all the muscles in the body including the muscles for breathing, we create a resistance free environment where we can easily intubate without inducing the gag reflex. Trying to intubate without paralysis is a difficult task: the patient often gags, yanks at the tube, turns their head, and even reflexively sits up. When intubating, we try to be as fast as possible to minimize the time the patient is without oxygen. This process is referred to as RSI, or rapid sequence intubation.

Dr. Rimelle had her instruments ready as we had practiced and now that Pauline was fully paralyzed, I instructed her to intubate per RSI protocol. She grasped her laryngoscope and locked it in position, making a characteristic clicking sound the scopes tend to make. I walked her through the process as she opened the mouth with her right hand and placed the cold steel with her left into Pauline's mouth. Sweeping the tongue to the side and out of the way, her windpipe was identified. A plastic tube was placed cleanly through and the metal removed. A bag with oxygen was connected and with that, her chest began to rise again. She was once again alive in the sense that she was breathing, albeit artificially. I listened to both lungs and determined the tube was in the correct location. The windpipe sits directly on top of the esophagus (tube to the stomach) and occasionally the tube is placed in the wrong location. After verification of correct placement we congratulated Dr. Rimelle and taped the tube in place. Our pharmacist readied medications to keep Pauline in a paralyzed state, thus allowing the seizures to stop and her brain to receive much needed oxygen. The paralytic and sedative medications we used to stop Pauline's seizures also kept her from breathing. We connected Pauline's breathing tube to the ventilator and took over the act of breathing for her.

Pauline was disrobed and ready for medical inspection. I assessed her from head to toe and found no obvious deformities other than her temperature, which was 103 degrees Fahrenheit. This could be from an underlying infection or from seizing so long. When seizing for a long time, the body naturally creates heat. As the muscles contract and relax (and sometimes stay contracted) energy is burned and heat is released. If this goes on for a long period of time the core body temperature itself can rise, leading to a fever. I listened to her lungs and could hear the harsh sounds of air being forced into and out by our ventilator. Her heart rate was regular and strong. Having been in status epilepticus for so long there was serious concern for brain damage and I wasn't sure if there was much left up top.

I shone my light in her pupils to see if they would shrink, a brain stem reflex. Normally a light shone in the pupils causes them to constrict. Her pupils did not respond. They remained fixed and dilated, an ominous sign. This meant her basic brain stem reflex wasn't working, suggesting extensive brain injury. Once she was stabilized, connected to the ventilator, and labs drawn she was moved to the ICU. Limited blood tests were sent and I performed a lumbar tap, taking some of her spinal fluid that surrounds the brain out to send to the lab for inspection for infection. While awaiting the results she was started on antibiotics. We took a CT scan of her head which showed diffuse areas of hypoxic brain injury, meaning a large portion of her brain had been without oxygen long enough that damage was evident on imaging.

The translators came to me with the parents and began reciting the history and slowly the pieces of the puzzle came together. Pauline had a fever for a few days prior. The second day of the fever her parents thought it was benign and treated her with local homeopathic remedies. They fed her soup of a local herb and tinctures they purchased from the local homeopathic provider. On the fourth day the fever did not subside and she began complaining to her parents that she had a headache and was feeling more and more tired. That evening her parents found her in the bedroom seizing. They did not know how long she had been seizing. The last time they saw her was an hour prior. They rushed her to the local homeopathic provider who gave her more tinctures and herbs. Over the course of that night the homeopathic provider worked endlessly to try and stop her seizing and fever. What began as two seizures in 3 hours turned into a seizure every 30 minutes and finally a nonstop whole body shaking. At this point the homeopathic provider realized this was out of his control and told the parents Pauline's "mind is dancing," and that they would need to go to the city to get treatment immediately. At six the following morning her parents straddled Pauline on a scooter and drove three hours to arrive at MSF Belgium's hospital in Port-Au-Prince. The entire time Pauline had been dancing.

Pauline was very sick and I needed help. I located Dr. Egger, a neurologist from New York, and asked him to opine on Pauline's case. I found Dr. Egger outside by the gate drinking a Coke. He was in his usual disheveled self; shirt half tucked in, pocket protector in place with at least 5 more pens then he needed, and glasses with tape holding the lens on the left in place with the frame as well as in the middle across the nose bridge. We tend to have stereotypical characteristics for most specialties in medicine: The cowboy Jack-of-All trades family physician (me), the jock orthopedist, and the Jeopardy-ish history buff random fact generator Infectious Disease specialist. The neurologist is the medical school nerd - often one of the smartest of the group and also the most socially challenged. He looked like he stepped out of a 1960's cartoon, the epitome of the neurologist nerd. I had grown fond of Dr. Egger – funny, nerdy, and a thoughtful and caring physician always willing to help in any way he could. I grabbed him and walked to the ER while briefing him on the situation. Dr. Egger evaluated Pauline and came to the same dire conclusion – it seemed her seizures had lasted so long that it likely damaged her brain. Still, she was young and healthy prior to all this and we both agreed she had a slight chance at recovery. We now had a team working on Pauline.

---

Later in the day Pauline's lab results were back and we huddled together as a team around her CT scan with various bits of information trying to come up with an explanation. Her lumbar tap showed that she likely had a viral infection. I had placed spinal fluid in 4 different tubes to avoid contamination and each of the four tubes agreed. We arrived at the logical conclusion that she had Herpes Simplex Virus Encephalitis – a viral infection of the brain. Her story fit. High fevers, no evidence of bacterial infection on her lumbar tap or elsewhere, new onset seizures that are difficult to control, and all at a young age. We knew the prognosis for this was poor to begin with but to make things worse, this was Haiti and Pauline had been seizing and infected for some time now. As we formulated a treatment plan, a major roadblock began to present itself.

Herpes encephalitis is treated with intravenous antiviral medications such as acyclovir. Up until now all Pauline had gotten were antibiotics, which only work to kill bacteria, not viruses. Essentially we had not given the child the medication she needed to try and slow the infection. IV Acyclovir is a difficult medication to come by and we had none in our pharmacy. For the next hour we called numerous hospitals and NGOs asking if anyone had intravenous acyclovir. No one had any in stock. Finally we collected about $100 USD from our team of volunteers and gave the money to the Father, telling him to go to every pharmacy and hospital in the area and try to buy some. Reluctantly he left on what seemed to me a wild goose chase. I knew finding intravenous acyclovir would be akin to finding gold in Haiti. What to do in the meantime? We improvised.

Our pharmacist found oral acyclovir in the pharmacy. Oral acyclovir isn't that strong and is usually used for more benign viral infections such as chicken pox, shingles, or genital/oral herpes. When taking an oral medication, there are many steps in its absorption. First of all part of the pill or powder will go straight through the gastro-intestinal tract, not being absorbed. The part that does get absorbed from the stomach then passes through the liver, our body's filter. Here, many drugs go through the 'First Pass Effect' where some of it is cleared away by the liver and some finally making it into the blood stream. Only a certain percentage of what you ingest actually gets put to use, what we call bio-availability. With intravenous medications on the other hand, the bio-availability is high with no first pass effect. That is, IV meds skip filtering by the stomach and liver. Meds given by IV are more potent than their oral counterparts. The cowboy, the nerd, and the pharmacist powwowed and after some research and calculations we came up with a fairly impressive plan.

144                                                                 *Dance Of The Mind*

We referenced the bio-availability of acyclovir which was thirty percent – meaning if we wanted 300 mg of active acyclovir in her blood to fight the infection, we had to give her 1500 mg orally. The average dose for a 250 pound man of oral acyclovir was no more than 800 mg two or three times a day. Pauline, weighing in at no more than fifty pounds, was going to receive 1500 mg every eight hours. We decided this was our last shot at saving the poor girl and placed a naso-gastric tube – tube going through her nose into her stomach – allowing us to give her the acyclovir. Nine hours, 3000mg and two doses of acyclovir later the roosters welcomed the sun back up and Father with it.

It was the break of dawn and Father returned empty handed. He had spent the entire night tirelessly roaming Port-Au-Prince stopping at every hospital and pharmacy that was open trying to find gold. He was exhausted. He had not slept in almost three days, eaten next to nothing, and held his spirits high as Haitian men did the entire time. He was a strong man who had lived a difficult life. Father was a farmer and he and Mother had a family of eight children who helped with their sorghum farm outside of the city. Most of their children were in their teen years but Pauline was the youngest and the most adored. She was the child who everyone worked to see succeed. Pauline was to go to school, college, and make a name for herself and her family. She was bright, witty, curious, and always loving. Father recollected one story in particular:

*Pauline was six and I was working a long day on the farm. It was Pauline's birthday. She was supposed to be in school but wanted nothing more than to spend the day with me. So we agreed her birthday present would be spending the day off from school. I asked her what she wanted to do that day and she said just watch me work. I spent all day farming and Pauline followed me around everywhere I went. When I picked up a shovel, she picked up a stick and mimicked me. When I pushed the sorghum roots in the ground, she did the same. She was my mirror image.*

*It was lunch time and my wife brought my food out for me. I usually come indoors to eat but today was a special day. We had a picnic outside and Pauline was happy as can be. I knew I did not have a lot to offer her for her birthday but she never complained. She was just happy to spend her day with me, Mother, and the rest of the family. We are a poor and simple family and family is the only wealth I have.*

*That is my Pauline.*

To see Pauline in this state devastated him; tube down her nose, breathing by a machine, lines coming out of her arms, and all the while Pauline's dance had not stopped. It would slow as the medications worked but soon after each dose, the dance came back. It was never as grand as it had been when she was admitted and now took on a subtlety. Her entire body lay still except for her right shoulder which would twitch upwards as if trying to shoo a fly away. This tic would occur regularly every five seconds or so, almost as if it were synchronized by a metronome. After many hours and a few doses of acyclovir, she was still having subtle seizures.

Dr. Egger and I re-evaluated Pauline and found no change in her status. Her pupils were still non-reactive to light, a repeat CT scan showed worsening swelling of the brain, and Pauline was not breathing on her own. We continued to call throughout the day in search of intravenous acyclovir but our gold was never to be found. As the day progressed Pauline did not recover. Her temperature would not come below 101 degrees Fahrenheit and her subtle seizures would not abate. Care was finally futile. She presented to us far too late and far too sick for treatment. We began discussing how to present the scenario to the parents to consider withdrawing care. There wasn't anything left we could do for her and she was using precious resources. We had 4 ventilators at the time, more than any other public hospital in PaP, and were always fielding requests for transfers to our hospital. At this point I had one ventilator available for an acute trauma if it came in, but if there were two, one would just have to die.

In our medical school training we all take a course on medical ethics or review topics during some of our learning sessions. One of the classic medical ethics scenarios involves utilization of limited resources, and another, medical futility.

*Utilization of limited resources scenario:* Imagine you are the physician on call in an emergency room when 3 cases of rattlesnake bite come in; a seven year old child, a 30 year old ex-felon turned preacher, and a 65 year old retired teacher. You check with your pharmacy and come to realize that there are only 2 doses of anti-venom. Without the anti-venom, one person will surely die. Who will get the anti-venom and survive and who will perish?

*Medical futility defined:* Medical interventions that may not provide any significant benefit to the patient.

*Medical futility scenario:* Imagine one of your elderly nursing home patients is admitted to the intensive care unit for a flare up of severe lung disease. She is hooked up to a ventilator to breathe and multiple attempts to wean ventilation over the next few days prove unsuccessful. She remains unresponsive due to the necessary sedation to provide mechanical ventilation. You and the other members of the medical team confirm that she would not be able to survive outside of the ICU. The patient's family requests that she stay on the ventilator. What do you do?

Scenarios like this, albeit an extreme, do occur and I now found myself in exactly such a situation. With one available ventilator I could only accommodate one new patient. Being the most equipped public trauma center it was only a matter of time until all our vents were needed. When another patient came in, how would I be able to justify keeping Pauline futilely connected when another had a chance of making it out alive? I knew the answer to that question – we would have to disconnect Pauline from the ventilator since at this point medical care had become futile *and* resources were limited here in PaP. We discussed this as a team and agreed to have a family meeting that night.

With parents at bedside we began the conversation. Conversations such as these (withdrawal of care) are difficult in-and-of themselves; add a language barrier and non-medical trained interpreters to the mix and one can imagine how difficult it was. Our translators work

*Dance Of The Mind*

hard but don't have formal training in medical translation. I can't even imagine how terms like 'encephalitis', 'swelling in the brain', 'seizing too long', 'irreversible brain damage', and 'medically futile' were translated. We answered a few questions father and mother had and went over the details of the case. After a few minutes they both confirmed they understood the gravity of the situation. We then discussed the real decision that had to be made: withdrawal of care. Parents understood that once we stopped the medications and took out the breathing tube Pauline would once again physically start seizing. The electrical activity in the brain was disorganized and our efforts at restoring it had failed. In her mind, she probably never stopped dancing. Once the breathing tube was removed, depending on how bad her brain stem was damaged, she would either stop breathing immediately or soon after and die. During this entire discussion, both parents stood quietly at Pauline's bedside, stroking her hair and nodding in agreement. After a long 30 second pause father said "Can we let her go in the morning?" To which we agreed – praying that we would have no patients that night that needed a ventilator.

---

Later that night Pauline's heart finally gave out. With extensive brain damage and no conductor left at the helm to lead her body through this ordeal she was not revivable. Pauline died with her Mother and Father at her bedside. The dancing had finally stopped. We left the family alone for a few hours.

In the morning Father asked us for money to help pay for the transport of the body back home and funeral costs. He asked with such humility it made me cry. We all could see how difficult it was for him to deal with the loss but to be humiliated by poverty was unbearable. Transport and funeral costs in Haiti came to about $500 USD which we were able to procure. Father and Mother took their darling Pauline in their arms and loaded into a vehicle and left.

Poverty had gotten the better of this family as it has of many around the world. Had Pauline been close to and taken to a competent physician and hospital when the seizure first occurred, she most likely would have survived this whole ordeal. Here in Haiti though, Pauline died.

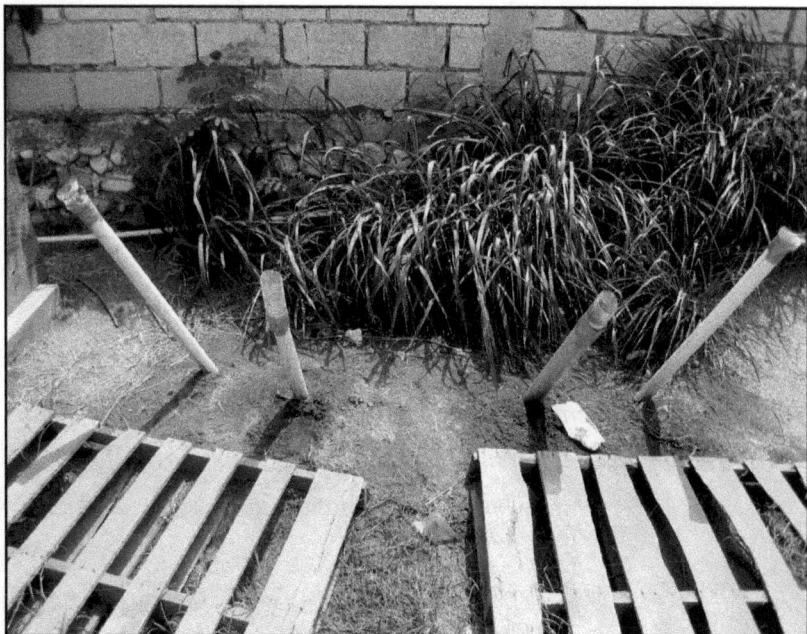

Men's urinals in the tent hospital.  Like a game, we would just point and shoot.

# Kissing Emily

*Death is the liberator of him whom freedom cannot release, the physician of him whom medicine cannot cure, and the comforter of him whom time cannot console.*

- Charles Caleb Colton -

# 9-1-1

The number 9-1-1 was established in 1967 in The United States. On average there are 240 million calls to 9-1-1, and 99 percent of the population in the U.S. is covered by 9-1-1 services. Have you ever stopped to think about how privileged we are for our emergency services? When we hear an ambulance whizzing by we pull our car to the side, thinking nothing of this luxury. If we have a medical emergency in most metropolitan regions in the United States, we can call 9-1-1 and have an ambulance there within minutes. The professional medics who come to our assistance can identify and stabilize the situation and transport us to a hospital for further care. Our system saves lives.

In many other countries emergency medical services are not given the urgency they receive in the United States. In India, for example, I watched cars sluggishly move over so that ambulances blaring their sirens could pass through downtown Bangalore. Some cars refused to move over while others would just speed up and move in front of the ambulance to get to where they were going. In Haiti emergency medical services are a luxury granted only to the minority who can hire their own ambulances. Police vehicles in Haiti oftentimes end up becoming patient transports and ambulances. The Police Nationale d'Haïti (PNH) can be found on every second or third block of metropolitan PaP. They mostly patrol the streets and provide an omnipresent existence. Common ambulances are sport-utility vehicles such as the Toyota Land Cruiser with their rear seats ripped out to allow a stretcher to be pulled in. There are a few true ambulances reserved mostly for private patients and paid hospital transport.

In Haiti it can take up to an hour to have an ambulance respond to an emergency. Civilians or the police become the primary mode of transportation for emergencies. Most of the time police place the injured person in the bed of their truck and shuttle over as fast as traffic allows. As a matter of fact, I remember one evening the police pulled in with a young male in the back of their truck. I hopped aboard to evaluate the scenario and immediately knew what I was dealing with. As I was taking in the scene the police officer explained through an interpreter that the young man was a fellow police officer who was stabbed in an altercation. "Did they do anything for him en route?" I asked the translator. The answer was as I expected, *no*. He was dead on arrival (DOA). He slowly bled to death on the one hour drive through PaP traffic. No one had provided even the most rudimentary of first aid skills – pressure to the wound to slow bleeding. Given the location and type of wound he may have survived with appropriate basic emergency medical care, starting with simply applying pressure at the source of the bleeding. Sad for him his colleagues did not have basic first aid training to stabilize the situation. This is the emergency medical transport system for most Haitians. Those of us who are fortunate enough to live in countries where emergency medical services are functioning need to be grateful for where our taxes go.

# Hematemesis

On average the human body has about five liters of blood flowing through it at any time. Blood is our life force – it carries nutrients and oxygen throughout our body and removes toxins and carbon dioxide. Before we knew what fire was, we surely knew that blood was crucial to our existence. If we were injured and bled and the bleeding was not controlled, we would die. It was as simple as that for our ancestors. Through the ages we have engrained the importance of blood in our genetics. Some of us feel faint at the sight of blood. After a paper cut many of us suck the blood from our fingers rather than wiping it away – quite an odd behavior indeed. We do not want to lose any of our life force, even a few precious drops.

Blood loss from a finger wound is one thing but throwing blood up, hematemesis, is another. Hematemesis is quite a scary word. It is derived from the Latin *heme* for "blood" and *emesis* for "vomiting." It can be from a torn blood vessel in the throat or lungs, a bad nosebleed, or even a ruptured ulcer in the upper gastrointestinal (GI) tract. We can lose significant amounts of blood through hematemesis in minutes and die just as fast. Bottom line, hematemesis is a medical emergency until proven otherwise.

## Emily

I was told an emergency was at the gate, so I grabbed my gloves, put my stethoscope around my neck, and went outside with my nurse. Inside our gate was the familiar white-and-blue PNH truck I have seen more times than I prefer. I saw the police escorting a young girl in her school uniform off the truck. She was hysterical, screaming and crying. She kept pointing to someone else in the back of the truck as she was escorted off. I instructed my translator to interrogate the girl and find out everything he could about what happened. I fought my way through the crowd gathered around the back of the truck and hopped in the bed. While climbing up I felt a wet, warm liquid against my gloves. I looked down and was astonished. The entire bed of the truck was covered in bright red blood. I saw two old tires and next to them lay a beautiful young Haitian schoolgirl, Emily, who looked to be around seventeen years old. Her immaculate French school uniform was stained red with blood. She lay limp and lifeless in between the tires. Those tires are made from oil, which is the end product of carbon degradation. Basically oil comes from old dead things like dinosaurs and other animals. Sadly, she had as little life left in her as those tires next to her in the bed of that cold steel truck. I quickly listened to her heart and lungs and verified she still had a mild pulse and shallow breathing – she was on the brink of death. Immediately we transported her into the ER and I began my assessment.

The story I was told started the morning on her way to school. The young girl was with her friend, and as majority of Haitians do, they took a *tap tap*. A *tap tap* is a colorful Haitian public transport. Essentially it's a privately owned pickup truck outfitted with benches. These vehicles are painted in vibrant busy colors of reds, greens, blues, and often have sayings and montages decorating them. These cabs transport people along set routes for a small amount of money. When they arrived at school both students were exiting the *tap tap*

156                                                              *Kissing Emily*

when Emily signaled to her friend for assistance. As Emily exited she grabbed her friend's shoulder and began vomiting. She vomited cups of dark, thick crimson blood. She knelt down and began vomiting again. This time she vomited bright red blood four or five times in a row, finally collapsing and fainting. Her immaculate white shirt which she ironed every morning at 6 at the behest of the mother turned red from the flow of blood. As she lay in a pool of her own life force, the police were flagged down and they put her in the back of the truck and drove her over. En route she vomited blood three more times. The police officers said initially she was in and out of consciousness. She would wake for a few seconds, say her chest and head hurt, vomit blood and faint again. After her third vomitus she did not regain consciousness and lay limp like a rag doll in the truck for the duration of the trip, about ten minutes.

Once I had her in the ER we checked her vital signs. Normally when people lose a large volume of blood their blood pressure drops and in response the body increases the heart rate to keep blood flowing to the vital organs. Her blood pressure was low but not dangerously so and her heart rate was within normal limits. For a brief instant I thought she might actually do okay. She was breathing on her own but taking very shallow breaths. Like a well-oiled machine our team smoothly got to work putting in IVs and starting IV fluids. A couple of minutes later as we were finishing up our initial evaluation she stopped breathing. Her electrocardiogram showed asystole (a flat line with no activity). Her heart had stopped beating. Immediately I signaled for the team to start CPR and asked for the airway and emergency code cart to be readied.

A code cart is a storage cart on wheels that holds an external defibrillator, emergency medications and supplies such as tubes and scopes to intubate. I called out for a few medications to get her heart to start beating again. She received epinephrine (adrenaline) and atropine which helped her regain a strong heart rate. I was in the zone – sweat dripped down my face, and my game face was on. This was a turning moment in this girl's life. No matter how many times I have faced this situation in the past, each and every time is heart wrenching and anxiety provoking. This girl's life was hanging by a thin thread and it was my job to ensure that this thread did not break. With this reality I prepared to intubate and provide mechanical ventilation for her.

Given the dire situation, she needed a tube put down her throat to help her breathe. The process of doing this is called intubation. I asked the team to stop CPR so I could intubate her. I lifted her chin and opened her mouth and received a direct whiff of blood. The smell of blood is unique – earthy with an iron undertone. Recall the last time you had a nosebleed? The taste and smell of blood never quite leaves your memory. As I opened her mouth the smell of fresh blood rushed in my nose and mouth, putting a deep iron like taste in the back of my throat. All I could see was a pool of blood in the back of her throat. I could not identify her trachea (tube to her lungs) or esophagus (tube to the stomach). I tried to suction out the blood. Our suction machine decided to stop working at the one crucial moment it was needed most. Frustrated, I placed a gauze sponge in the back of her throat to absorb some of the blood. After a few frustrating tries we finally had her intubated. We connected her to oxygen and were now breathing for her. I rechecked her pulse and her heartbeat had come back strong; we had stabilized her, for now.

I had her basic labs sent off, IV fluids running in her veins, we were breathing for her, and we had heart rate back. At this point I still had no idea what caused her to nearly die. Generally speaking, I had a working differential diagnosis but needed some more basic information such as a chest X-ray and labs. Ideally, as in the United States, a patient like this would have received an emergent CT (computed tomography) scan, an endoscopy (camera down the esophagus and stomach), and bronchoscopy (camera down her trachea) to find the source of bleeding. Thus far I didn't even have an X-ray! We did not have a portable X-ray machine so I would have to take her about sixty yards away to the radiology room. I decided we needed to take this risk since the X-ray might help piece together this puzzle. The X-ray would also help confirm placement of the breathing tube in the right location. I asked our very competent clinical pharmacist to go ahead of us with the code cart. We wheeled her over to the radiology suite and as we were getting ready to shoot her X-rays, her pulse slowly became faint. After a few seconds it was completely gone. I couldn't feel it! The portable monitor still showed an electrical rhythm, but without a palpable pulse her heart was essentially not pumping – a condition known as pulseless electrical activity (PEA). We resumed CPR and she received more medications to kick-start her heart. After four minutes of CPR her pulse came back and we took the X-rays and wheeled her directly to the ICU.

The breathing tube was in the right place but her X-rays showed she had a pneumothorax on the left side (air in between the lung and chest where it shouldn't be) and a hydro- or hemothorax on the right side (fluid or blood between the lung and chest where it shouldn't be). After stabilizing her in the ICU we got to work on her lungs. With the guidance of an excellent critical care physician I put a needle in Emily's left chest. Since there was air built up, the needle would allow the air to escape. A loud *whoooosssshhhhhh* came from the needle as air rapidly deflated from the chest cavity. After that a tube was inserted into the chest space to relieve the pressure and allow the lung to re-expand and do its job. We then placed another tube on the right chest to get rid of the fluid and help the lung expand.

Up to this point Emily had been extremely lucky and blessed. She arrived basically dead in the back of a dirty police truck. As she clung to life we worked our hardest with our limited resources to bring her back and were successful. Yet without finding the source of her bleeding we knew she was at risk of bleeding to death at any moment. I called our medical director, who informed me that an endoscopy would not be a possibility until the next day at the minimum. She also needed a camera put down her breathing tube, a procedure called bronchoscopy. I inquired into this and was told bronchoscopy was a total no go. Apparently there are only a couple of bronchoscopes in PaP and they cost a fortune to use – reserved for the wealthy. We had a pulmonary physician with us, but no bronchoscope for him to use. Bronchoscopes are pulmonary physicians' tools of the trade; much like a hammer is to a contractor, a bronchoscope is to every pulmonist. Nothing was more frustrating than knowing we had the expert but not the tool he needed to save Emily's life. "I've got 3 bronchoscopes sitting around my office that I don't even use. If I knew we didn't have any down here I would have brought one to donate," the pulmonist said. It was a cruel irony.

In the United States, a patient losing blood will get emergency blood transfusions to keep the blood level at a minimum safe level. This was not the United States. We had one unit of emergency blood which took three hours to obtain. To get more blood we had to send Emily's family members to the Red Cross to donate blood in a sort of 1 to 1 exchange. Due to the critical shortage of blood, the Red Cross in PaP works on an exchange system: donate blood to receive blood. A few hours later Emily's mother had made it to the hospital. She sent other family members to the Red Cross to donate/bring back blood. Emily remained stable overnight. She was ventilated and received copious amounts of IV fluids. Her chest tubes continued to drain fluid. In the morning Emily's family returned with 2 units of blood which we immediately transfused into Emily. Prior to receiving blood, her blood level (hemoglobin) was 6.8 (normal is 13).

Later that day she received her endoscopy – well...sort of. In the United States, an endoscopy is done by a gastroenterologist, a physician who is trained in diseases of the GI (gastrointestinal – stomach and intestines) tract. Again, this was not the United States. The physician who came, Dr. Ante, was a local Haitian generalist who happened to have an interest in GI medicine. He was trained in general adult medicine but did not do any formal specialty training in GI medicine. He had taken it on himself to learn how to perform endoscopies and colonoscopies and purchased is own scopes. He was short, balding, and spoke no English. Even though I couldn't understand what he was saying, I felt his humility. He was soft-spoken and exuded an aura of seniority and calm. He did not have an endoscope but did have a colonoscope (camera that goes up the colon). These cameras are similar in function but the colonoscope does not have all the features the endoscope does, such as the ability to close a bleeding blood vessel. Nonetheless, that was all he had so he put the colonoscope down her mouth.

Dr. Ante was trying to locate the source of bleeding. If it was in her stomach or esophagus, he should be able to find it with the camera. He spent an adequate amount of time searching but was unable to find any bleeding and withdrew his scope. This left us frustrated beyond words. Where was she bleeding from? It was from one of two places: her trachea and lungs (respiratory tract) or her esophagus and stomach (GI tract). If the blood had been coming from her respiratory tract we surely would have seen blood in her lungs, which we did not see on X-ray. If the blood had been coming from her GI tract we should have been able to see the source on endoscopy, which we did not. I wondered if Dr. Ante had been able to visualize her entire upper GI tract with the colonoscope. I was frustrated but satisfied I had stabilized her up to this point. We still had no idea how long her brain had gone without blood. Would she ever wake up? Was she going to have any remaining brain function? Was all of this medical care futile? Why did this all happen? Would she live in this resource-limited country for long? Either way, she was stable now and we had to think about what to do next.

## Extubation

Children and young adults are resilient. Had a sixty-year-old man gone through the bleeding and cardiopulmonary arrests Emily had, he most likely would not have survived. Kids seem to snap back like rubber bands.

Emily lay there intubated and ventilated. During ventilation a machine is pushing air in and out of the lungs artificially. One can imagine how uncomfortable this would be if a patient was awake; hence we try to keep patients sedated during ventilation. Over time we slowly wean off the medications and test the patient's respiratory status. Two days later Emily's labs had stabilized and she was no longer bleeding. When we would lower her sedative medications she would become agitated; moving her arms and legs, moaning, and trying to pull at her tube. As we weaned off the medicine, Emily surprised us all. She awoke agitated. This was an excellent sign! It meant her brain was still working and she was ready for a trial of extubation (taking the breathing tube out). We still didn't know the cause but she at least seemed to be stable and recovering rather well.

A couple of hours later we told the mother about our plan to extubate. As the medications wore off we verified Emily was alert. She nodded her head in response to our instructions and questions. We told her what to expect as we took the tube out and she acknowledged this. The tape was removed from her tube and the tube was quickly pulled out. She gagged and coughed as patients always do when the tube is removed. It took her a minute or two to stabilize her breathing and resume the act of completely breathing for herself. Her voice was hoarse, irritated by the tube but completely normal. A successful extubation! It was a great day.

Emily smiled and responded to our voices a few minutes after the tube was removed. She slowly regained her voice, albeit raspy and thanked us for our work. I slowly got to learn who Emily was. She was a quiet but smart student. She wanted to go to college and become a nurse or doctor. Shy, she never made eye contact for more than a few seconds with me. Her smile, however, told it all. Every time I would walk in the room her face would light up and her smile thanked me and the team for what we had done. She had come a long way and she knew it. Emily understood she had nearly died. As she lay there in bed I noticed something in her eyes. Outside she seemed happy and giggly. Inside she was still scared. Scared of what had happened and what might happen next. There was a deep thought hidden in her eyes. Something I hadn't seen before. Her eyes seemed to hold a secret, something she had not shared with me. *What could it be?* I wondered.

When I left for dinner Emily was tired and took a nap. She had enough excitement for the day and after losing as much blood as she did, her body was showing signs of fatigue. The physician covering the ICU told me later that as soon as I left Emily's respiratory status worsened. She was working harder to breathe and tiring out very easily. Her lungs and heart were fatigued. The stress of breathing was too much for her right now. In medicine, night is the proverbial shadow – death lurks in the night and we try our best to avoid risky situations during that time. Since it was still evening and there was a full staff present, the physician taking care of her decided to re-intubate Emily for safety. Essentially the plan was to give her body a break and let the machine breathe for her overnight. The intubation went well and the next morning she was extubated again. Emily had no further episodes of bleeding and remained stable the next day – awake, alert, smiling, but scared.

## The Kiss

Saturday came. It was time for me to begin my voyage home and leave Haiti once again. I could not have asked for a better day. I awoke as usual to my phone alarm at 0630. I began my morning ritual by eating a few bites to wake up my bowels. As long as I eat a few bites in the morning, my gastro-colic reflex works like clockwork. The food entering my stomach stimulates nerves in the lower colon to make room, causing a bowel movement. Like a finely tuned machine, every morning I take a few bites, have a bowel movement, brush my teeth with bottled water and follow it up with a shower.

Showers are short and sweet. Our water is limited and cold, brought in by a truck every day. I turned on the faucet and a trickle of cold water fell from the showerhead. I am used to the water wasting warm Niagara Falls of showerheads back home. The drop-by-drop cold-water trickle is always the worst part of the day in Haiti. As the cold water hits my head, I shiver and shake it off. *Whatever you do, don't drink the water ... keep your mouth closed*, I tell myself as I wash. The tap water here is filled with parasites waiting for an opportunity to invade and attack my GI tract and cause diarrhea. I quickly lather and condition my hair. My entire shower is done in less than two minutes.

I clothed up, finished packing all my gear, and packed a suitcase full of my supplies to donate: sleeping bag, mosquito net, soap, body wipes, food, etc. This suitcase would make its way to a few of the millions in need here in Haiti. *Where is my shampoo?* I wondered. It was missing in the shower today. I would find out later at the airport that one of my Canadian colleagues had an eye for my Head & Shoulders and packed it away in her bag to take home. However, she packed it in her carry-on and when she was going through security at the airport later that day it was found and discarded. To this day, I tease her for swiping my shampoo! She mailed me a couple bottles of maple syrup to make up for it. That was fine with me – I'm a maple syrup connoisseur and nobody makes maple syrup like the Canadians. I wonder if they have Head & Shoulder's in Canada. My next adventure in life is to set up an import export business to Canada with my Canadian friend: import maple syrup and export Head & Shoulders.

After readying myself I grabbed my medical bag and walked over to the ER. Albeit we were leaving today the new team would not arrive until noon; thus we were scheduled to work until 1 PM at which time we would sign out our unit and head to the airport. Walking over to the ER I looked around and appreciated the sites I saw. It would be a few months until I'd be back and I knew I'd miss it. To my left was the same juvenile rooster I saw combing the hospital grounds daily. Every morning he and a few other young chickens would run around searching for food. I had no idea who they actually belonged to but they lived on campus just like us. Looking at the young stud as I walked by I knew today was the last day I would see him before he ended up as someone's meal. He acknowledged me and continued searching for breakfast as I smiled and walked past him into the ER. Entering the ER I received a clean sign out, meaning my beds were empty so I did not have to take over anyone else's patients.

My day in the ER was uneventful; a couple of minor issues and lacerations came in. I began saying my goodbyes to the staff and friends I had made. As we exchanged e-mails, Facebook info, and phone numbers with one another I had one goal on my agenda I could not pass up. I had promised my medical team that if we kept Emily alive, I would give her a kiss before we left. It was now our day of departure and Emily was awake, alert, breathing on her own, and speaking. We saved Emily's life. She came in the back of a truck basically dead and we saved her – a true miracle. I prepared myself to kiss Emily goodbye.

I wondered what all of this must feel like for her. Imagine being seventeen again and on your way to school you start vomiting blood; the next thing you recall is waking in a strange setting. It is hard to breathe; you feel like gagging, something is in your throat. You try taking a big breath in but something is shoving air into your lungs. *Wait, I didn't take a breath, what's pushing air in me?* The force of a ventilator pushing air in your lungs is overwhelming. As you start to become agitated, you slowly open your eyes and look around and see white walls and blurry figures rushing around. A slow hum begins to enter your hearing followed by a musical chime from the ventilator and a beep that seems to happen at a constant fixed interval. The sounds are almost orchestral, but at the level of an unorganized elementary school band. What begins as hushed whispers amplifies into alien jargon. You cannot understand what is being said around you but you know people are talking and scurrying about. You fall asleep. You wake up a few more times and, at one point, feel like throwing up as something is being pulled out of your throat. You are scared and as you become more agitated, you hear a voice. One of the blurry fleeting images is now in front of you and slowly coming into focus. You hear the words "You are in the hospital, relax and take in deep breaths." Slowly it all comes back: *I was throwing up blood and now I must be in a hospital.* You focus on the person standing next to you and it is your mom. Relieved, you start crying and listen closely as your story over the past four days is told back to you. As you listen you slowly understand your situation and why half the staff around you are not Haitian and speaking in foreign tongues; you are in a hospital run by foreigners. You finally put all the pieces of the puzzle together and feel a bit more secure. Just then a bearded dark-skinned foreigner who speaks English comes up and kisses you – likely the scariest part of the whole ordeal!

Luckily I had prepared Emily for my smooch. Like a chivalrous knight after saving her life, I respectfully asked her mother for her permission. "Would it be okay if I gave your daughter a kiss goodbye and take a picture to remember her by?" I asked. Her mother gleefully agreed. I then asked Emily the same question and she shyly

168                                              *Kissing Emily*

smiled and nodded her head in agreement. I handed my camera to a friend to photograph this moment. Emily was sitting up in her bed, holding a cup of water. Her hair was done up, almost ready for this moment. He mother had combed her weave and styled it, as if she were going to prom. She looked alive again.

I stood next to her and smiled; she smiled back, not making eye contact for more than a second before she timidly looked down, all the time still smiling. Her immaculate white teeth, symmetric high-riding cheekbones, and dimples made her look like a teen beauty queen. The photographer signaled he was ready and I leaned over and kissed Emily on the forehead. I felt the warmth of her skin against my lips, and that half second felt like a lifetime. I could smell and taste the sweat from her body which had been washed numerous times with body wipes, leaving a hint of alcohol in the background. I saw her skin; dark and smooth as it glistened under the fluorescent lighting of the ICU. As I stood there, the noises in the room faded out and all I could hear was Emily. Not Emily's physical calling, voice, or her heartbeat, but rather first the silence of the room followed by the presence of her being. In that moment, I felt her soul; I felt the life that was fleeting, which I grabbed ahold of and pulled back into her. I felt her thanking me. I felt her thanking God silently for the time she was given to see her mother, tell her how much she loved her. In that silence, she said her goodbye to me and I to her. This moment of intimacy was shared only by Emily, me, and God. At that moment I *knew* Emily and she *knew* me. I had saved Emily and given her a kiss goodbye.

As physicians, we play intimate roles in the lives of patients. When I touch a patient, I listen to the story the body is telling me. Even though disrobed, my patient is still covered from me. The skin and organs hide inside them their story, and it is my job to interpret it. Resting the stethoscope gently against the chest, I listen to the story the heart and lungs tell me. Other than the stethoscope, it is the direct skin-to-skin contact between physician and patient through which crucial information is had. A skilled physician is a master of all his senses: tactile, feeling the story the body has to tell; smell and taste intertwined, breathing in all the body has to say, we use our throat and palate to taste the patient's life; sound, listening to the tale the body is repeating over and over in its own rhythm; and vision, with my eyes, I am scanning the body looking for clues and signs. In no other situation other than love would a consenting individual disrobe themselves and willfully allow you to experience their body. This bodily communication is what truly differentiates a scientist from a physician. The basic science is learned easily and stored in the brain, but interpreting a human body is the art of medicine.

## Stupid Facebook

I said my formal salutations to Emily and her mother and was on my way. It was four days later when I finally got around to loading my images on my computer. As I looked at the picture of our kiss, something caught my attention. Emily's eyes were open and she was looking deeply beyond the camera. Staring at her photo I noticed that her eyes seemed shallow. Not shallow in a superficial physical sense, but shallow in a more ephemeral sense. Her eyes reminded me about the secret I felt she had hidden before. Her eyes burned into my soul, telling me what I already knew but refused to acknowledge. She had a secret she was keeping, but her eyes were giving it away. How could I have not seen this before? Maybe I had seen it but knew there was nothing I could do about it. Emily told this secret to me in our kiss as well, but I refused to listen. The physician in me had interpreted what she was telling me but the person in me ignored it.

I already knew what was coming before I opened my Facebook that day. I had been in contact with a friend/nurse who was in Haiti for another week. In a Facebook message she wrote:

*She got intubated late Saturday night and was just not doing well. Monday afternoon we proned her [changed positions] and she seemed to like it but was still sick. She coded 3 times Tuesday night before they stopped. The new docs aren't as good as you guys were. It was a pretty rough day. I'm sorry.*

Her eyes in that photograph had burned into my soul. I had done everything I could in such a resource-limited setting to save Emily's life. Had we been in the United States, she likely would have survived, but this was Haiti. I fought bravely for Emily as her knight in shining armor and valiantly left her with an intimate kiss. No matter what we did Emily had to die and she knew this. Somehow when death nears, many know their time is coming. I'm sure Emily knew. In the end, God had already called for Emily and my role in her life story was not to save her physical vessel. Rather, I had bought Emily precious time to spend with her mother. To say her goodbyes and make peace with this world – something many people aren't lucky enough to have. In her eyes she had come to terms with this. She knew she was going to die and she had told me this during our kiss. I didn't want to believe it and ignored it.

I will never forget my Emily and my gallant fight to save her. Now it is my turn to come to terms with her passing. Patients are people and so are doctors. When we take care of patients we often befriend them. We put in countless hours, energy, and effort in caring for our patients. When a patient of mine dies, I've lost a friend. It is never easy losing a patient, and each and every day I carry a bit of my patients with me. Emily is with me every day and she constantly tells me I did my job, but it is still hard to come to terms with it. In a way, I feel like I failed as a doctor. I questioned the different decisions that were made. I found myself blaming the doctors that took over my place and her care. In the end, it was her time to go and nothing we as doctors could have done to save her. I can at least walk away from the situation knowing that I brought her much-needed precious time. Time to say goodbye and time to express love to her family – a blessing many don't get – and left the poverty of Haiti and the suffering of this world behind for a better place.

## Dr. Ante

Finding a specialist in Haiti who is willing to work with the poor populace we serve is always a difficult task. Many physicians leave the country after their education. The few that remain receive differing levels of education. Specialty training is difficult to obtain and often without an objective unanimous curriculum, thus yielding physicians with various levels of knowledge and training.

172                                                         *Kissing Emily*

A few months later on a subsequent trip I would again consult Dr. Ante for an urgent endoscopy on a patient. We transported the patient to his office where he performed the procedure. In the United States, an endoscopy is done under light sedation. It is quite uncomfortable to have a tube pushed down the esophagus, eliciting the gag reflex constantly. Dr. Ante offered sedation to patients who could afford to pay for it. In his clinic procedure room he had a gas machine ready to deliver the sedative gas. My patient, however, could not afford to pay thus he performed the entire procedure sans sedation and she was in incredible discomfort throughout. Stoic as most Haitians are, she sat as still as she could during the procedure while gagging, coughing, and tearing from pain. Dr. Ante was doing the best with what he had, and in his mind sedation was a luxury not a necessity.

At the end of the procedure he diagnosed her with chronic gastritis, or long standing inflammation of the lining stomach. Gastritis is treated by medications and avoidance of triggers such as certain medications (ibuprofen, naproxen, and aspirin), alcohol, caffeine, spicy foods, greasy foods, smoking, and stress. After writing up a brief report Dr. Ante told me she had chronic gastritis and recommended nothing except an aspirin daily for the pain. I was taken aback. The mantra of gastritis treatment which even those not in the medical field can recite is 'no aspirin for patients with gastritis.' I asked him to repeat his recommendation and he once again said the same. Appalled, I thanked him for his time, took the patients report and left. On the ambulance ride back to our hospital I crossed out his recommendation from the report so the patient wouldn't see it at another time and actually try aspirin to treat her gastritis.

How could such a basic fact as this be wrongly recommended? Luckily for my patient I was there to help correct the misinformation. But what if I had not been there? This bothered me greatly. It's one thing to not know something, but to give information that can actually harm a patient was scary. Part of the Hippocratic Oath states (in Latin) "Primum non nocere," translated "First, do no harm." Although Dr. Ante meant no harm of course, had she taken his advice to add an aspirin daily, the gastritis may have turned into a bleeding ulcer and led to death.

I still don't know why Dr. Ante recommended an aspirin for gastritis but I commend him for his willingness to work with our patients. I don't know if the hospital pays him a stipend for being available for our patients. Whether or not they do, he could be seeing private patients during that time and making much more. Doctors like Dr. Ante are limited in Haiti. Few doctors are willing to donate time and resources to the underserved. This isn't a problem that plagues Haiti alone. All around the world many physicians practice medicine as a hobby or business, not as a social duty. Here in the U.S. the number of new physicians willing to work with the underserved and work in primary care (preventative medicine) is waning. New graduates would rather work in a private setting as a specialist making 3-10 times what an underserved primary care provider would make. This is a complex problem with many reasons, one of the biggest driving factors being medical school debt. The average medical school graduation debt is $165,000 - $205,000. With such debt looming overhead it's becoming harder and harder to convince graduates to enter underserved primary care. Worldwide we are faced with a shortage of doctors whose job is to keep patients healthy. Instead we have a flux of specialist ready to fix a broken problem. Apple wouldn't cut its design engineers in half and hire double the repair technicians would they? They see the value in investing in preventative engineering to prevent problems later down the road. So why don't we invest more in preventative medicine? Why wait till it's broke? A complex problem indeed with a complex solution we are working on. While we work on fixing this disparity, we do the best with what little we have. In the meantime, patients continue to get sick and lack access to care here in the U.S., Haiti, and all around the world.

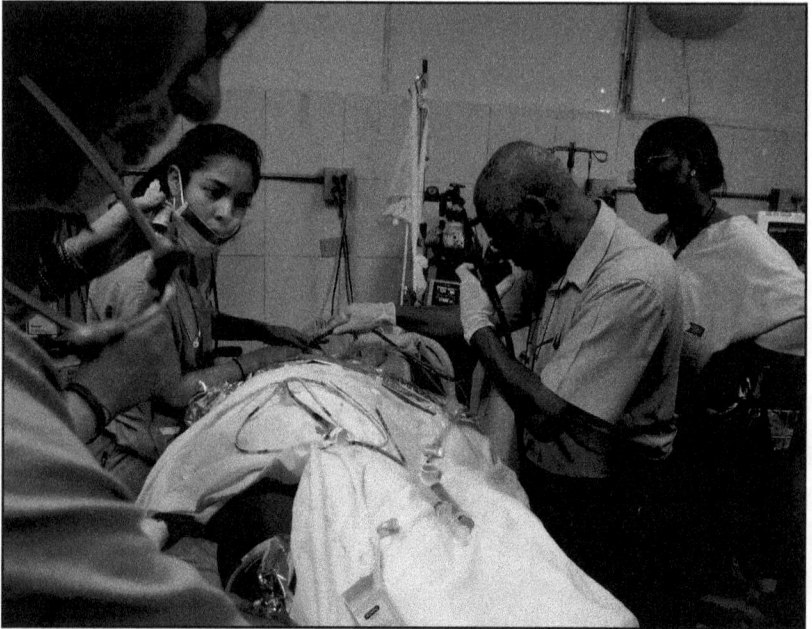

Haitian doctor looking down a patient's stomach with a camera (endoscopy) designed to be used for looking up the rectum (colonoscopy).

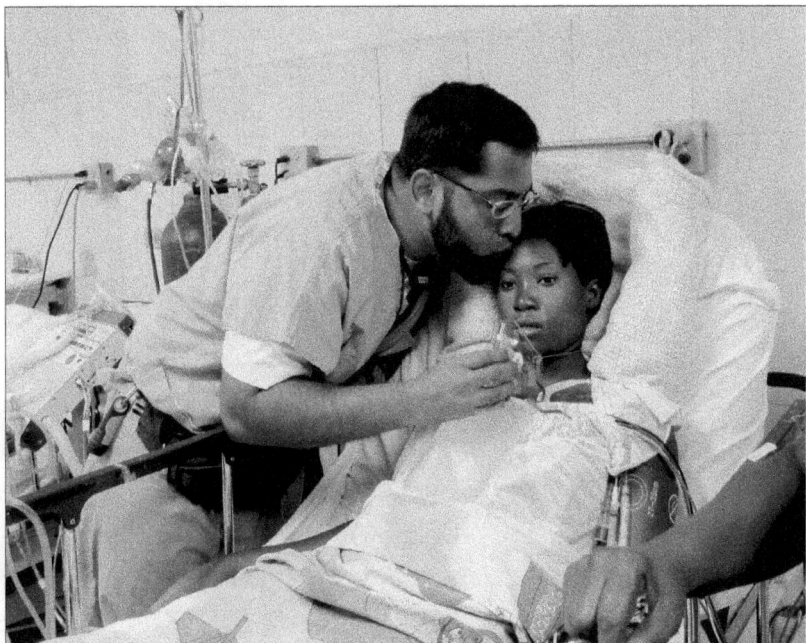

Emily the day I left her.
(Picture used with permission of Emily's Mother)

# Life Goes on

*Life is simple, it's just not easy.*

- Unknown -

*Forgive, O Lord, my little jokes on Thee,*
*And I'll forgive Thy great big one on me.*

- Robert Frost -

If there was one word to describe Haitians it would be resilient. Through decades of poverty, war, famine, disease, natural disasters, and political instability Haitians have learned to adapt and quickly move forward with their lives. One Haitian, Mary, summarized it to me as "Why stay sad so long? We just be happy and move on." And move on they did. Soon after the earthquake I was surprised to see people jogging on the streets, business men going to work in suits, street vendors and shops pawning their respective goods. Where an event like Hurricane Katrina brought New Orleans and much of the region to a standstill (even areas that weren't flooded), Haitians had learned to "be happy and move on."

## Karine's Call for Help

Mary was a beautiful young woman in her mid-twenties. She lived in Bonga, a rural city in Southern Haiti. Bonga is a hilly paradise about a three hour drive from PaP. Green rolling hills encompass the landscape. Tropical vegetation and trees grow abundantly as far as the eye can see. Far enough from the main coast, the humidity and temperature are more tolerable than many other parts of Haiti. Less inhabited, running water, electricity, and sewage are luxuries out of reach for most in this area.

Mary and her husband worked and lived on her parents' farm. Hundreds of years ago their family was stolen from West Africa and brought as slaves to farm tobacco as were most African Haitians. Over the generations she and her extended family stayed close to the area. For some time the families tried farming sugar cane but eventually returned to tobacco. With time, many family members moved to

PaP or other cities. Those that stayed continued the family's legacy of tobacco farming. A few decades ago their tobacco leaves were purchased by some of the major cigar and cigarette companies in Haiti and the Dominican Republic. Although cigarette use is on the decline around the world, cigar smoking tends to hold steady. They still sell their tobacco leaves to cigar manufacturers.

Cuban cigars, of course, are world renowned for their flavor and quality. Given the long standing trade embargo, many cigar companies have found other ways to export Cuban quality cigars to the countries such as the U.S. Companies grow Cuban tobacco seeds in other temperate countries including the Dominican Republic and Haiti. These leaves are then dried, processed, and rolled into cigars which are in turn sold as "Cuban Origin" cigars which are legally exported to Cuban trade embargoed countries. For the past twenty years or so Mary's family has been involved in the cigar tobacco industry which has been lucrative enough to allow for a fairly humble but stable rural lifestyle including electricity.

As a young girl in rural Haiti, formal education was a luxury she would not see. She stayed in school long enough to learn how to read and write, and that's about it. On her plantation, Mary received an education of a different sort – education on life. She learned to seed, farm, cultivate, harvest, dry, and sell tobacco leaves along with household duties and chores. Over the years Mary's beauty blossomed and she was quite the teenager. Her mother warned her to keep fast to her chores and stay away from boys, especially her cousin Maxime, or Max. Max was two years older than Mary and they had known each other their entire lives. He was quite interested in Mary and spent most of his day working the farms with her. Ignoring her mother's advice, Mary enjoyed the time she spent with Max and kept it up. Eventually Max and Mary found and recognized their love for each other and were wed. She was fifteen and he seventeen. Within a few months Mary was pregnant with their first child, Odette. She had no formal prenatal care and was delivered by her aunt, a sort of midwife without the formal education. Six months later, Mary was pregnant again.

Initially her pregnancy was quite normal. Like her prior pregnancy with Odette, Mary continued to work the farms. She seeded and harvested tobacco plants through most of her term. Mary swore up and down that she wore gardening gloves whenever she worked to prevent tobacco exposure. When she was about 6 months pregnant her belly was big enough that bending and picking/planting was not possible and she retired to working mostly with leaf drying and packaging. Around 7 months into her pregnancy Mary began noticing a few symptoms she had not had in her prior pregnancy. She experienced vague dull headaches which seemed to come and go without any inciting factors. Her aunt, the midwife, gave her an herbal tea to drink which seemed to help for some time. However, after a few days the headaches returned and with a vengeance. The pain was a severe, vice like pain which started in the front of her head and moved towards the back. She described it like someone had put her brain on a "tobacco leave flattening roller." She drank more tea and hoped it would go away.

A few days later while taking off her shoes, Mary thought it funny that the shoes had left indentations on her feet. She knew to expect some edema (swelling) but not this rapidly nor this early. Over the next two days it became more and more difficult to put the shoes on. Her hands and feet were swollen and she just couldn't shake that nasty headache. She began seeing scotoma (spots in her vision) that she thought were because her headache was getting bad. At that point, her aunt realized the situation was more serious than she had originally thought. She called the local doctor over to have a look at Mary. Upon hearing the symptoms and evaluating Mary, the doctor was rightly concerned and said she needed to see an obstetrician at a local hospital. He thought she had pre-eclampsia, a serious disease.

The local hospital was an hour drive away. Max knew it would cost a good amount of money just to be seen there let alone the cost of any treatments or procedures needed. From past experiences he knew the doctors wouldn't provide said treatments unless the patient paid up front and purchased the required medications. Although they were not the poorest family in Bonga, a large hospital bill would be something he wouldn't be able to afford on his own. Max did not want to burden Mary's family with such costs either. He had a friend who had moved to PaP shortly after the earthquake to work as a translator for international organizations. His friend had recently gotten a job at a hospital called Project Medishare on the grounds of the airport. Max went to the local grocery store and used their phone to ring his friend, Widson. Widson told Max that he knew one of the doctors at the hospital fairly well and suggested he bring Mary to the hospital that night while he was working.

Hesitant about leaving, Mary agreed to Max's plan. Mary had spent most of her life in Bonga. She had travelled to PaP a few times only to be under impressed and overwhelmed. Leaving her comfort zone was difficult. They packed a bag with a few clothes and mounted onto Max's 2-stroke Chinese made motorcycle. It was still early in the day and they planned to reach PaP by the evening before dark. As they drove, Mary thought of the risk they were taking by leaving the security of their home. PaP was a large, dirty, and scary city. After the earthquake she had heard that the rate of violent crimes had increased in and around the city, especially in the slums and surrounding tent cities. Scared, Mary knew she had to go. Her headaches became more intense and the spots in her vision more common. She no longer fit into her shoes and had to wear sandals. Her hands were so swollen that her wedding ring caused her constant pain; she finally removed the ring and left it at home. A few hours later with no valuables other than their motorcycle Max and Mary safely arrived in PaP and found Widson.

Widson was born and raised in Haiti. He studied English in school, fascinated by the thought of a better life in the U.S. His parents owned land and were financially well off enough to allow him to pursue his studies in English. In his late teen years he illegally immigrated to Houston. He worked and saved money for three years for his journey to Houston. First he flew from PaP to Mexico City then took a bus to Nuevo Laredo. There he found a coyote (human smuggler) that was willing to smuggle him into the U.S. for $2500. He was driven to Hidalgo, a small city at the Texas-Mexico border. At night they boarded a raft and illegally crossed over the Rio Grande River, the natural border between The U.S. and Mexico. From there he was shuttled to Crystal City, Texas where his uncle received him.

After a few weeks in Crystal City Widson moved to Houston where he worked delivering pizzas during the daytime and parking cars at night. He found a girlfriend and had a child. Life was good. Four years later while waiting for the bus to take him to work he got into an argument with someone. Words led to pushing which led to a fight. Police arrived and detained both individuals. Widson had a driver's license but no proof of citizenship or permanent resident status and was subsequently found to be an illegal immigrant. Without any regard to the family or life he had built, he was quickly deported back to Haiti.

In Haiti he worked odd jobs for two years until the earthquake struck. Soon after the quake he realized the potential job opportunities for translators and moved to PaP and eventually ended up with Project Medishare. I met Widson on my first tour to Haiti and had worked with him on subsequent trips. Bright, motivated, and eager to learn Widson created his own dictionary of words that he carried with him. The dictionary wasn't limited to English words, but contained phrases and words in numerous languages. Any time he met a foreign worker he picked up a few phrases. His dictionary contained expressions in English, German, Spanish, Hindi, Arabic, and even Cantonese. I quickly learned to respect his thirst for knowledge. In another world, perhaps one in which he was born into a privileged Haitian family or in an industrialized nation, he may have been a

*Life Goes On*

professor or academician.

Widson approached me to tell me about his friend Max and Mary. I was the only physician practicing obstetrics at the hospital and was on call every night during that week. I was covering the ER and OB that day. Widson proceeded to brief me on the history of the case. Intrigued by Mary's history, I told Widson to bring them both into the ER and inform me personally when they arrived. A couple of hours later Widson found me and told me they were waiting.

At first glance Mary appeared normal, hands at her side and sitting straight up. Once I put my hands on her I knew she was sick. As I examined her the problem became more obvious. Her fingers were swollen and looked like sausages ready to burst. Her feet and legs were also swollen. She complained of a nagging headache and spots in her vision. I immediately checked her blood pressure and found it to be highly abnormal, elevated at 180(systolic)/105(diastolic); normal being less than 140/90. A urine test showed her kidneys were leaking large amounts of protein. Mary had severe pre-eclampsia, a very serious and potentially life threatening illness of pregnancy.

---

Pre-eclampsia (formally known as toxemia) is a serious condition in pregnancy which is defined by two criteria: high blood pressures and significant amounts of protein in the urine. It is thought the maternal body builds an immune response against the placenta and fights it off as an intruder. The cause is not fully understood but what we do know is the placenta becomes sick during this disease and secretes different factors into the blood. These factors cause the blood pressure to elevate, growth restriction in the baby, kidney damage in the mother, and can progress to a more severe disease called eclampsia.

Eclampsia is the above plus seizures and can lead to bleeding in the brain of the mother and death. Pre-eclampsia can be mild or severe, based on symptoms and/or blood pressures and/or the amount of protein in the urine. Mild pre-eclampsia can be delivered in most cases in 1-2 days. There is a saying in obstetrics: "Never let the sun set on a severe pre-eclamptic." Meaning a severe pre-eclamptic should be delivered as soon as possible and within 24 hours of induction to prevent progression to eclampsia. Eclamptic patients need to be stabilized and delivered immediately.

The only known cure for pre-eclampsia is removal of the offending agent, the placenta. That means to treat this disease we have to get the baby delivered, either by vaginal delivery or cesarean section. Most cases of pre-eclampsia occur towards the latter part of pregnancy so delivering the baby a few weeks early is acceptable. It does, however, also occur earlier in the pregnancy called early onset pre-eclampsia, and has worse outcomes. If the patient is a severe pre-eclamptic and far from the due date, even though the fetus may not be ready for delivery the fetus needs to be delivered to save both mom and fetus's life. Studies have shown that the closer to the due date the delivery occurs, the less cognitive delay later in life for the child. Also, a fetus's lungs develop during the middle and latter portion of the third trimester. The earlier a fetus is delivered from its due date, the higher the likelihood of lung or brain development problems. We try to hasten delivery on mild pre-eclamptics as long as possible but expedite delivery of severe pre-eclamptic or eclamptic patients.

To prevent some of the pre-term complications when delivered early we intervene with certain medications for the fetus' development. If the mother's blood pressure can tolerate waiting 1-2 days, we will inject her with a steroid such as betamethasone. The steroid helps create an enzyme in the lung to give the fetus a better chance at breathing on its own when delivered. We provide a medication to the mother called magnesium: this medication helps prevent contractions and slow the labor to give time for the steroids to reach the baby and work. It also has been shown in studies to assist brain development in the fetus. Lastly, magnesium helps prevent seizures and thus is a crucial part of the treatment. These mediations, when given in utero if the mother is not a severe pre-eclamptic or has progressed to eclampsia, give the fetus a good fighting chance when it is delivered pre-term and keep the mother stable and safe in the interim.

Magnesium is usually given intravenously via slow infusion to prevent unwanted sequalae (side effects) such as lung and heart problems. Physicians trained fifteen or twenty years ago did not have IV pumps and administered magnesium via intramuscular injections every 4 hours or so in the buttocks. With the advent of IV pumps this method was sent to the wayside as its efficacy varied dose to dose, location to location, and patient to patient. IV pumps provided a more definitive and objective delivery of a potentially dangerous medication. Younger physicians from medically advanced systems are not familiar with intramuscular delivery of magnesium and are dependent on IV pumps – that was me.

During administration of magnesium and labor the fetus needs to be monitored continuously. As the placenta is attacked by the immune cells more and more, it is weakened. Since this is the life line for the fetus connecting it to its blood and nutrient supply, maintenance of adequate placental blood flow is crucial to the survival of the fetus. The first warning sign the placenta may be finally giving out is decelerations, or drops in the fetal heart rate. Thus we continually monitor the fetal heart rate to ensure the fetus is tolerating the laboring process.

Mary was a severe pre-eclamptic, preterm at 33 weeks, and needed to be delivered soon. Albeit we did not have betamethasone available, there was another type of steroid which we began administering to aid fetal lung maturity. I ordered magnesium infusion like I usually do back in the States, not knowing we had no IV pump. A few minutes later the nurse told me she searched everywhere in the hospital and could not find the appropriate pump for magnesium. I was stumped. How was I going to give her the magnesium she so needed? Luckily a quick internet search with the query 'old way to give magnesium in pre-eclampsia' gave me my answer. I found the World Health Organization (WHO) guidelines and read through them. Following their instructions I began giving her shots of magnesium in her buttocks and medicine in her veins to lower her blood pressure. I gave her shots of oxytocin, a hormonal medication that causes contractions to induce her labor. To top it all off, we had no form of continuous fetal monitoring. The best I could do was use a fetal Doppler intermittently. A fetal Doppler is a small machine unit which has a probe that can be placed on the abdomen to listen to the fetal heart rate. The heart rate is then calculated manually. It is essentially a stethoscope to listen to the fetus, which of course cannot be done continuously. Every fifteen minutes or so when I wasn't busy I came over to listen to the fetal heart rate for a minute or so and then went back to work.

I closely watched the clock and hoped the oxytocin would induce her labor and my medications would keep her pre-eclampsia controlled. Even though she wasn't formally educated, Mary was quite intelligent and understood the gravity of the situation – and this made her and Max very scared. As the day progressed her blood pressures worsened, creeping up to the severe range numerous times. Even after receiving intravenous blood pressure lowering medications her pressure would rebound to values as high as 190/110. The lowest I could get her blood pressure was 155/100 and that only lasted a few minutes. To top it all off, I had no continuous fetal heart rate monitoring and this scared me.

Later in the day her blood pressures hadn't come down and she had two values that were 190/110. With the oxytocin on board and working, she was contracting every 6 minutes and feeling the strength of each contraction getting stronger. Prior to starting the oxytocin I had placed a small balloon in the cervix (opening to the uterus) to try and dilate it. I rechecked her cervix and found it to be the exact same dilation. Even with the oxytocin and balloon she had not moved forward in her labor. It had been twelve hours since her admission; her blood pressures were dangerously high and her cervix wasn't opening. Mary said her headache was coming back.

I routinely put my Doppler on her abdomen to check the fetus's heart rate as I had been doing every half hour for a few minutes. I found it and it was a healthy 130. As I listened for a minute I noticed it began dipping: 130...120...110...100...95...90. A fetus's normal heart rate is anywhere from 110-160, but mostly in the 130's. 90, albeit a normal heart rate for an adult, is a dangerously low heart rate for a fetus, analogous to a heart rate of 40 in an adult. With a low heart rate, toxins cannot be appropriately cleared from the blood and the fetus does not receive adequate oxygenation. A few short and intermittent decelerations in the heart rate a fetus can tolerate. Prolonged decelerations (more than two minutes) it cannot. Toxins build up and the fetus becomes acidotic and can die.

I tried the standard interventions: she as getting more IV fluids, we put her on oxygen, and we had her flip on different sides to see if that would help. Two minutes later the fetal heart rate was still in the 90's. At that point I knew we were in trouble. The pre-eclampsia had severely affected the placenta and the fetus was showing signs of decompensating. If we did not get this fetus delivered immediately both Mary and the fetus could die.

I told one of the nurses to grab Chung the anesthesiologist, Paula the pediatrician, and John a surgical resident as an assistant for an emergent cesarean section. I explained the situation to Mary and

Max as we urgently wheeled her to the tent next door where the operating room was. Mary cried and asked if her baby would die. No, I told her as I squeezed her hand. I glanced up and saw tears welt up in Max's eyes. We entered the OR and I asked Max to wait outside. Mary was quickly placed on the operating table as Chung and John arrived, both half asleep. I had completely lost track of time and forgot it was 3 in the morning. I placed the Doppler on Mary's abdomen and listened to the heart rate, still in the 90's. I verified that it wasn't mom by checking her pulse, 70. We are taught in obstetrics ideally to have a baby delivered within 10 minutes of a prolonged deceleration. It had been 8 minutes and the baby was still in the 90's. As Chung hurriedly put her under general anesthesia, John and I scrubbed and donned our surgical gowns and gloves. 14 minutes.

"Scalpel," I yelled. The Haitian scrub technician was still putting her gown on. I grabbed the blade and made a clean and decisive cut through the skin. I smoothly cut right through the fat down to the underlying layer of fascia (protective layer before the muscles and pelvic organs). The fascia glistened in the light of my headlamp. I sliced through the fascia, exposing the muscles. John and I inserted our fingers in the muscles and pulled in opposite directions, opening up the pelvic cavity. With my blade in hand I incised the uterus and opened up the incision. A window into the fetus's world opened and I could see the head inside the amniotic sac. Rupturing the amniotic sac, I placed my hand behind the fetus's head. John pushed on Mary's abdomen and I pulled the head, shoulders, and body out. Once out of the mother's protective womb, a fetus is graduated to infant status. We cut the cord that connected Mary to her fetus, and handed Mary's new infant to the pediatrician.

Paula evaluated the infant. She had come out limp and quiet. After what seemed like an eternity of resuscitation, Karine let out a loud cry. She was here and wanted everyone to know it. When I heard the cry I felt shivers down my spine. Certain things in life make everything I do worthwhile: the touch of my wife's soft skin, the smell of fresh rain, and the sound of a new life taking its first breath. We saved her. We closed Mary back up and within a few minutes were done. Paula was satisfied with Karine's health. I held Karine in my arms and walked to find Max sitting outside with his head buried deep in his hands.

As the doors opened Max raised his head and saw Karine for the first time. Only one word could define the look on Max's face, bliss. I handed her to him and told him whatever happens never let go of her, she's special. I told him Mary was going to be okay and would be brought out in a few minutes. Over the course of the next couple of days Mary's blood pressures normalized and on discharge her blood pressure was 115/60. The cure for her disease was actually quite simple; removal of the placenta. With the offending agent removed Mary was doing well. Overjoyed and relieved at the same time, our ordeal was finished. A few days later Mary and Max left for Bonga with the newest addition to their family, Karine.

Mothers and fetuses/infants die far too frequently in medically underserved nations from medical conditions like pre-eclampsia. Screening and prevention are key interventions but access to qualified

*Life Goes On*

expert care is also lacking. The few higher level care obstetrics hospitals in the area are overwhelmed and understaffed.

The physicians who work there do so in an almost superhero like fashion – every day with limited resources and an increasing patient panel. With adequate donations and time hopefully every hospital that manages obstetrics patients will have access to continuous electronic fetal monitoring and appropriate medications and their modality of delivery such as IV pumps. Until then, we do the best with what we have – and in this case, we heard Karine's cry for help just in time.

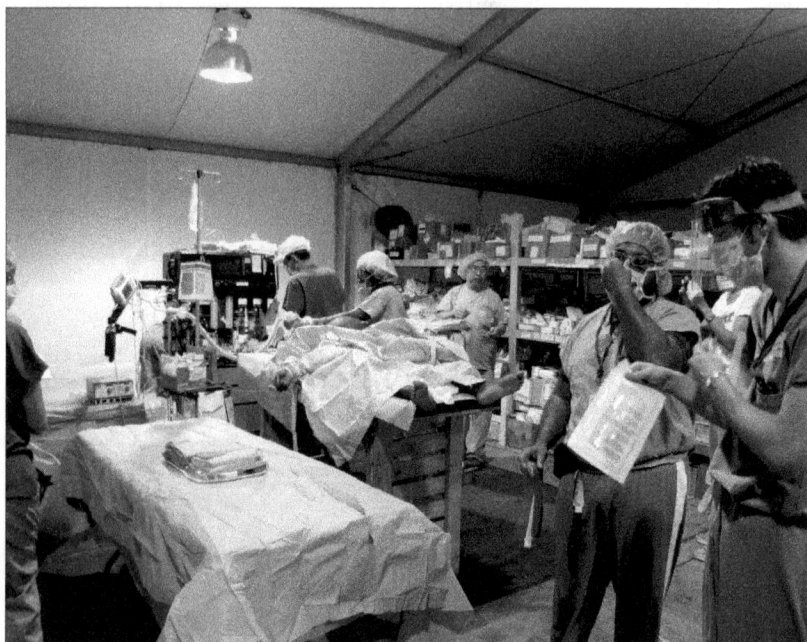
Operating room in the tent hospital. We prepare for an emergent cesarean section.

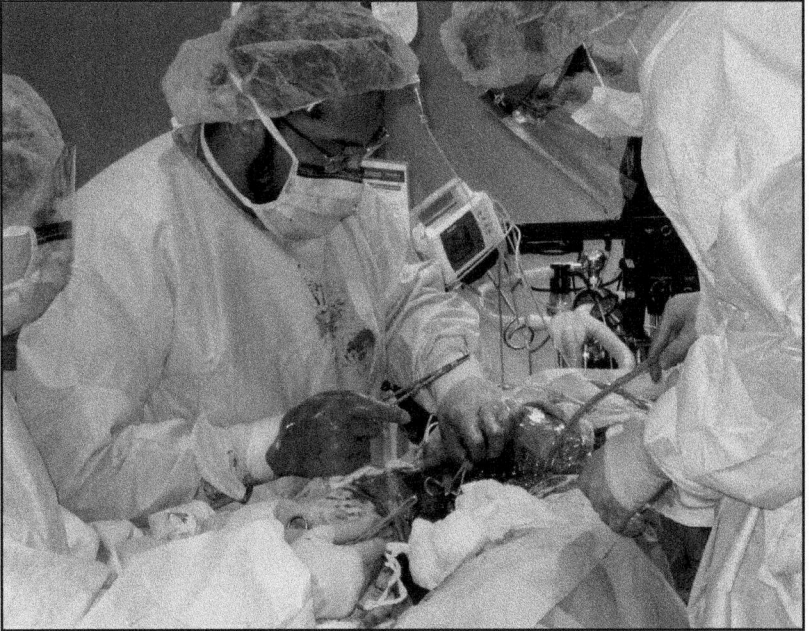

Performing an emergent cesarean section to save Karine's life.

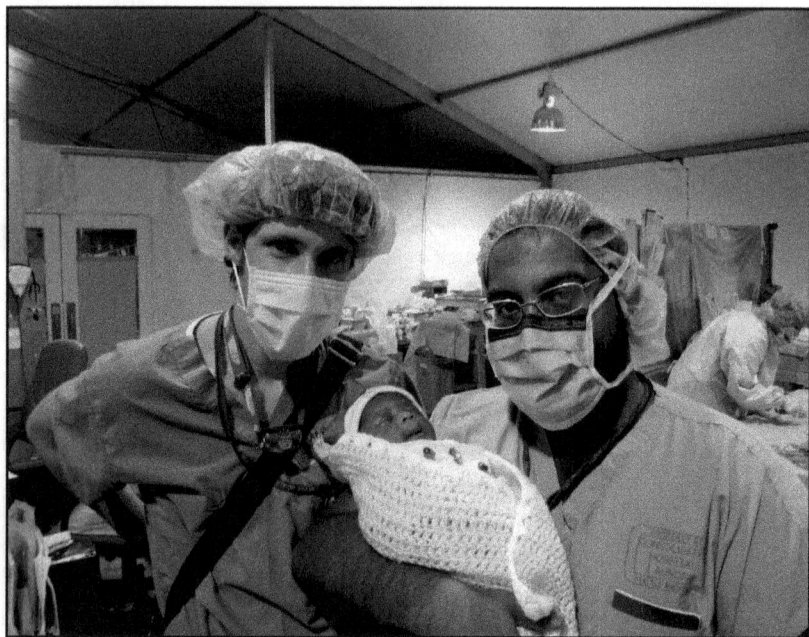

Karine, born from emergent cesarean section.

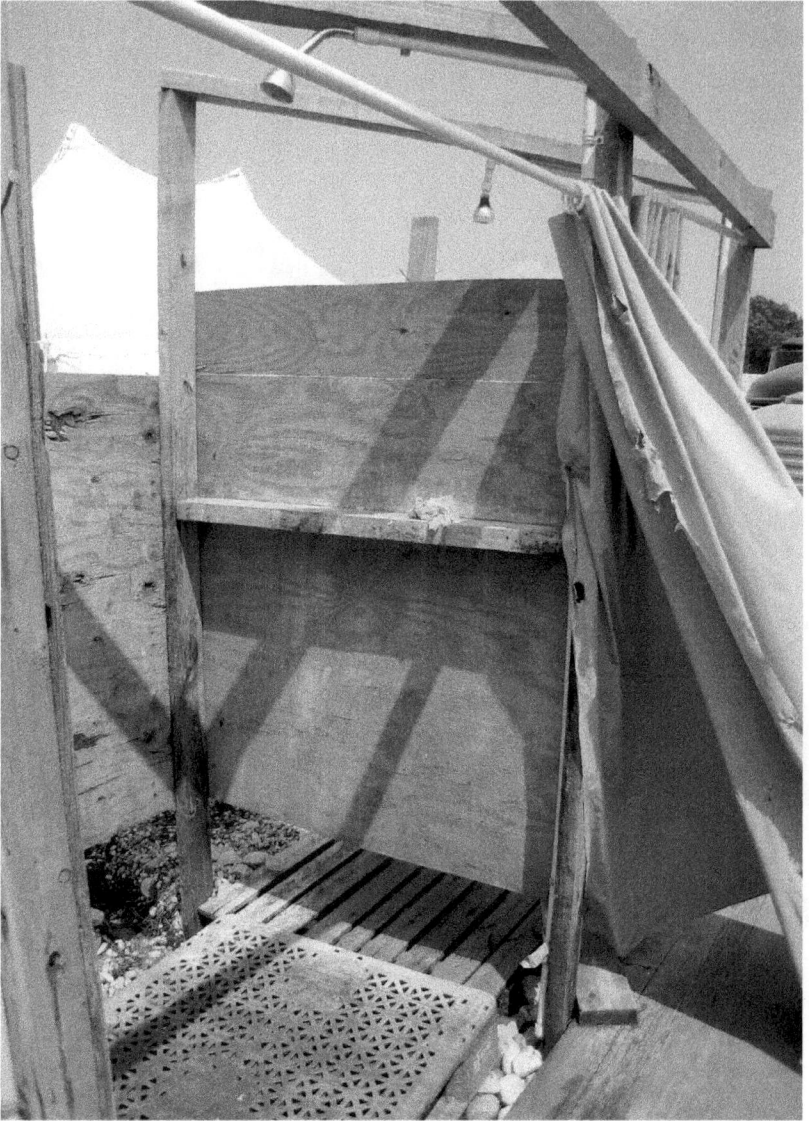

Our outside cold water showers.

# Taking Care of Ourselves

*A hero is a man who is afraid to run away.*

- English Proverb -

# The Beetle and the Leatherman

During the months our hospital was run on the grounds of the airport we tried to keep our tent operating room as clean and semi-sterile as possible. No matter how hard we tried it was never ideal. A few feet away from the tables the flaps of the tent were tied down to prevent things entering from outside. Every now and then a breeze would break through and carry dust and dirt into the OR.

Jim, a husky orthopedic surgeon from New York, was operating to change the hardware on a patient's leg when an unexpected visitor arrived. Completely scrubbed in, sterile, and in the middle of aligning the hardware he was fixing a beetle flew onto Jim's chest and landed there. He looked around and we were all laughing. "What do I do about this beetle," he asked - to which we had no answer. After pondering it for a few seconds he said, "Oh well, it's Haiti, even beetles are welcome in the OR. Maybe he can help me finish this case." With that the beetle took his cue and flew off Jim's gown. We laughed and he continued the procedure like nothing had happened. Had something like that occurred in the U.S. the entire sterile field would have to be re-sterilized and the procedure stopped. Then again, we wouldn't be operating out of a tent!

A day or two later Jim was unable to find a specific size screwdriver for an operation. After searching through our instrument kits he was about to give up when ingenuity kicked in. His Leatherman Multi-tool had an array of screw driver tips as one of the attachments. He found the size he needed and attached it to the Leatherman. He washed it thoroughly with antiseptic soap and put it in the autoclave machine to be sterilized. A few hours later, there he was in the operating room screwing closed a fixation device on a patient's leg with a $50 dollar Leatherman Multi-tool instead of the standard $1000 dollar or more medical screwdriver we are overcharged for – in the end the same outcome. Ingenuity goes a long way in Haiti. Lighthearted stories like these help keep us sane during the stress of international work. Laughing about a beetle or Leatherman helped keep us grounded and push away much of the sorrow we saw for a moment or two.

---

Volunteers had to be especially careful in caring for themselves. It was common to have a volunteer taking up one of the beds in the hospital recovering from dehydration or diarrhea. This was especially common during the months we operated as a tent hospital. Sweltering tropical heat coupled with the Caribbean humidity led to an almost constant state of sweating. After working an eight or twelve hour shift, one would lose liters of water in sweat. Keeping up with this rapid loss of water and salts was a full time job. When volunteers couldn't, they would be rehydrated with intravenous fluids and lay down for a few hours. Most of the time I took care of colleagues it was in this scenario – dehydration and fluid management. Occasionally the situation would be more concerning.

# Dengue

Liz was a Physician's Assistant from the U.S. who had been volunteering in Haiti for the past 6 months. Quite the accomplished practitioner, she had worked for numerous years before deciding to travel the world providing medical care. She had worked in Sudan for two years, India for 3, and now Haiti. Having been here for 3 months prior to the earthquake she experienced the disaster first hand. Liz was working with an international organization that helped provide basic medical care to orphans. She and her fiancй (a nurse) both decided to volunteer their time and travel around the globe providing medical care. Now they were in Haiti.

Liz came to our hospital complaining of generalized fatigue, weakness, severe pain in her muscles and joints, and a crushing headache. Over the past week she had progressively become weaker and unable to work an entire day. Yesterday she was so tired she slept all day and all night. Worried, her fiancй wanted her to be evaluated and brought her in. Liz endorsed having chills, sweats, and feeling febrile. At night she awoke drenched in sweat through to her covers. She knew something was wrong and thought she had malaria or typhoid, showing me numerous mosquito bites.

On evaluation Liz was severely dehydrated; her blood pressure was low, heart rate high, and her skin lacked the laxity a normally hydrated person would possess. Her temperature read 103° Fahrenheit yet she shivered violently. She had a severe form of shivering called rigors, which is an uncontrolled reaction of the body to her illness. Shivers are the body's mechanism of keeping warm. When cold, the muscles contract and relax rapidly releasing heat as they burn energy. Rigors, on the other hand, are an uncontrollable severe whole body shakes caused by the release of inflammatory agents during an infection. She described her eyes as feeling like a fire had been lit behind them. She moaned in pain from the rigors and fatigue. There was a spotted measles like rash on her skin. Out of the few illness that could make her this sick, the most likely culprit was Dengue Fever.

Dengue virus is a mosquito borne illness often seen in the Tropics and equatorial regions. Given the extreme joint and muscle pains experienced during the illness, Dengue has been commonly dubbed 'Break Back Fever.' There are different forms of Dengue and the first infection is usually self-resolving. Treatment consists of aggressive fluid hydration and pain management. Tylenol is used to keep the fever under control as well. Once infected with one type, the body is immune to that type of infection for the future. If infected by another subtype however, the second round of Dengue can be life threatening. The body overreacts to the infection and begins attacking its own cells. Cells responsible for coagulation (stopping bleeding) are broken down, leading to Dengue Hemorrhagic Fever. If not appropriately managed, patients can bleed from their IV sites, gums, and other orifices. When this continues unabated the organs are damaged, leading to the most dangerous form of the illness – Dengue Shock Syndrome. In Dengue Shock Syndrome the body is unable to combat the bleeding disorder and maintain adequate blood pressures. With time, these patients bleed from their eyes, nose, mouth, and eventually die.

*Taking Care Of Ourselves*

Even with the nighttime use of a mosquito net, Liz had been bitten by mosquitoes numerous times during her stay. There is no widely accepted laboratory diagnosis for Dengue and thus a combination of clinical findings, history, and laboratory results are used in combination to arrive at a diagnosis of Dengue. Her white blood cell count and platelets were both low. The lab findings along with the fine pin point rash I saw on her skin were concerning. Small blood vessels were breaking in the skin leaving that measles like rash. Her laboratory findings and history were consistent with Dengue Hemorrhagic Fever. Platelets are one of the body's natural glues, stopping bleeding from cuts and small vessels. If platelets are used up faster than the body can remake them, one can start bleeding from small blood vessels that rupture during the rigors. Turns out during one of Liz's trips to Sudan a few years back she had acquired a Dengue infection and had done well. This was at least the second time she had been infected with Dengue, putting her at risk for Dengue Hemorrhagic Fever and Shock Syndrome. She was stable at this point but I knew the situation could take a turn for the worse at any time.

I had read about Dengue numerous times but had only seen it once or twice. I had never seen Dengue Hemorrhagic fever and naturally questioned my diagnosis. Could this be something else like typhoid? I tried an old trick I remember reading about called the Tourniquet Test to confirm she had Hemorrhagic Fever. Placing a blood pressure cuff on her arm, I pumped it up tightly and watched her fingers and hand for a couple of minutes. This tests for fragility in small blood vessels, thus indirectly evaluating the coagulation system in resource poor settings where access to labs is not always an option. In a non-infected person with no bleeding problems, one should see few or no spots appear on the hands – signifying a working coagulation system. After a couple of minutes Liz's hands and fingers had multiple tiny red dots on them, called petechiae. Small blood vessels could not hold the failing blood products inside of them under the pressure of the cuff I had applied, causing the red spots to appear as these small vessels ruptured. Confirmed: Liz had Dengue Hemorrhagic Fever.

Liz received high doses of Tylenol every four hours, pain medication, and copious amounts of intravenous fluids. As always, obtaining blood products was next to impossible if she began to bleed. If she made it through the night without bleeding her fiancń had a plan to save her. They had purchased traveler's insurance and a medical evacuation was arranged for early in the morning. The plane was to take her directly to Miami for treatment.

That night I checked on Liz frequently. She tossed and turned in pain but made it through the night without bleeding or destabilizing into shock. Early the next morning a private ambulance picked Liz up and left for the airport. I would find out that one week later Liz was discharged from the hospital in Miami and had done quite well. She was preparing to return to Haiti to complete her unfinished work. Even 'Break Back Fever' couldn't stop this hero from returning to her mission to serve others.

---

Health hazards are one of the risks with international work, personal safety is another. Often times the political environment we enter is unstable or dangerous. For the most part we stayed on the hospital campus but there were times where we went abroad to other hospitals and clinics to help out. There were a couple of close calls. One excursion went quite well but the trip back was a bit more complicated.

I had staffed the outpatient clinic at The General Hospital for the day and was on my way home with a few colleagues. It was an exhausting day. I had seen over 300 patients out of a tent with only one working fan. It was a 90 degree day with high humidity and I had sweat off at least two pounds. Having only eaten a couple of protein bars all day, I was exhausted and hungry. I knew I still had to get back to our hospital and make rounds on my patients. Our tent hospital was on the airport at the time. We were in our private hospital vehicle when our driver pulled up to the gate to let us in. There was a longer and more hush-hush style conversation between the driver and the guard at the gate than usual. After a minute he turned the vehicle around and drove away from base. Surprised, we asked what was going on. The driver filled us in.

Turns out President Préval had gone to the United States for political fundraising and the airport management, knowing the President was away, thought it was time for a good ole fashion shake down. Up until now our hospital was running under the invitation of the President and his direct request to operate on the airport grounds.

With the President away, the airport management saw our hospital as a potential source of income. They had approached the hospital leadership demanding money, which they refused to give. Out of spite, the airport management put the hospital on lock down, allowing only Haitians to come and go. No international workers were allowed to enter or leave the airport premises, under the prudence of 'illegal visitation.' This was an immigration violation which would lead to arrest, or so the story was told to us.

Our team of volunteers had been off base while all this took place. The guard, offended by the situation, told the driver to turn around before his supervisor returned. Before sending us off the driver and guard had concocted an ingenious plan (the hush-hush part of their conversation). After turning the corner and getting out of site, the driver hailed down a colorful and overcrowded Tap Tap and told us to get in. Tap Taps are Haitian private taxi buses of sorts, brightly colored with images and photos of heroes drawn on them. They are the primary mode of transportation for the majority of Haitians. The Tap Tap stopped and we awkwardly boarded. There were four rows of chairs, all packed tight with Haitians. Some had chickens in their laps and others children. The whole bus had a stench of stale sweat which I fit right into. Recall that I had probably lost two or more pounds of water in sweat that day since there was no circulating air in the tent wards at the General Hospital. We each squeezed in between the Haitians and livestock. One in each row, we tried to blend in as much as possible: local Haitians on one side, a chicken on the other, and in between a foreigner with blue scrubs. I guess blend in isn't the right term after all since we so sorely stuck out.

*Taking Care Of Ourselves*

Our driver paid the Tap Tap driver and we were off. The same guard stood watch and hurriedly waved the Tap Tap on without once looking inside. Had there been any other guard and had they cared to look, I think finding a Haitian would have been harder than finding the foreigners in blue scrubs hiding in the Tap Tap. Through the gates we drove until we entered the hospital campus. The Tap Tap rolled to a rough halt and we, along with half the original passengers who so boldly helped keep us hidden, disembarked our Trojan horse. Ironically I would care for many of those passengers a few minutes later in the outside triage/clinic.

Looking back at it, the whole situation is laughable now; medical volunteers in blue and green scrubs trying to blend in with Haitians and livestock in a Tap Tap to sneak back into the airport hospital. Later that evening the lock down was resolved after hospital administration got a hold of personnel in Miami who phoned President Préval who in turn defused the situation by sending his staff to the airport. All was well once again ... for now.

---

One day while staffing The Police Clinic near the capital, a different type of danger presented itself. People had gathered outside the capital building to protest parliamentary elections. Over the course of a couple of hours, the size of the crowd had grown drastically. What started as a few people had now become a substantial gathering of a couple hundred. The window next to me was facing the main street. What I called a window was really just a large cut out of the wall. There was no glass, only a 3 foot by 3 foot opening to the street. I could hear the background noise as I worked; mumbling, an orchestrated hum, and chanting. The smell of street vendors and their goods constantly permeated the room throughout the day. Fried plantains and grilled meat stirred my senses. What started out as a background noise slowly escalated to a room filling protest chant. I could hear police sirens and yelling through a megaphone, which I interpreted as capital police telling the protesters to disperse.

Thinking nothing of it, I continued to do what I had come for. As I was evaluating a patient I heard screaming and yelling coming from the street. We both stood up and looked out the window. People were running away from the capital building, covering their faces with their shirts or blouses. As I took in the scene I heard a loud *thump* and looked down to see a canister spewing gas immediately below the window. It was a tear gas canister that had hit the wall and fallen right in front of my face. The police were firing tear gas canisters into the crowd to disperse them and had nearly hit me. I knew if it had hit me, the resulting damage could have been serious as they fall with a relatively high velocity from the firing arc. I had never seen tear gas canisters in action first hand and was surprised at the speed of gas dissemination.

Within a few seconds as I was still interpreting what was going on, a cloud of smoke was working its way into the room. I backed away and started coughing. My eyes felt like I had rubbed them after forgetting to wash my hands from cutting chili peppers. I could feel my lungs tighten as the chemical irritation kicked up my asthma. As the lungs tighten each breath becomes shallower. With less air coming in and less oxygenation occurring, the body's response is to breath faster to compensate, perpetuating an uncomfortable cycle of fast, shallow, ineffective breaths. It is hard to describe the feeling to those who have never experienced an asthma attack. The best analogy I have been able to come up with thus far is like being in space. Imagine taking in breaths but not getting in any air – a horrible feeling of suffocation began to overtake me. I could hear myself wheezing and dosed myself with the albuterol inhaler I always carried. I didn't use it often but knew the prudent thing to do was carry it on me when I left the base. My lungs responded to the medication and albeit I was still wheezing, I could breathe much easier.

Chuck, a fellow physician and an active soldier let his military training lead the way. He took control of the situation by yelling out commands. Following his instructions we lay on our abdomens and covered our faces with our shirts. Taking slow and steady breaths we crawled towards the exit at the other side of the room. As I crawled I noticed the straight lines of the tiles beneath me. I had never looked at tiles this close up before and noticed the porous structure. As I did, a cockroach scurried hurriedly in front of me. Was he following Chuck's instructions as well? I didn't want to know what else was on the floor I was so intimate with right now and decided to keep my eyes forward as I crawled.

My skin began to itch and burn as I crawled. It felt like someone had lit a match underneath. Remember those athlete's foot commercials? The one where they show a foot with a fire between the toes? That's what it felt like right now except my whole skin was involved - it was on fire. My eyes burned and I was coughing from the gas yet sneezing at the same time. I kept crawling. Once we reached the exit we stood up and walked towards the other side of the building. We found a sink and washed our face, eyes, and hands. Slowly, my eyes and skin stopped burning. I stopped coughing, crying and sneezing. My wheezing ceased and I was able to take in full breaths of air. Military tear gas is no joke! This isn't your wife's pepper spray. This is the real deal. I washed out my face for another 15 minutes.

My lungs were a bit tight and face irritated but overall I felt much better. Once the gas settled a couple of us went in and set up fans to blow out any residual. After about 30 minutes we moved back in and got right back to work. People who minutes before were outside protesting now came in as patients. Most of the complaints were due to the gas; skin irritation, tearing, coughing, and exacerbations of asthma. A few came in with heart palpitations from the excitement but all were cared for and left in good health. "Hey, a little tear gas never killed anybody," chuckled Chuck as we closed the clinic and went back to the base. *Yes it has*, I thought, happy that it wasn't me today. Severe asthma attacks when exposed to tear gas have killed many people in the past. Today I dodged that bullet.

## Big Dave

In a constant state of extreme poverty and neglect, many are forced to make desperate and often ill-fated decisions. On January 24th, 2012 Dave Bompart, an international volunteer, was robbed and shot. He was at a bank withdrawing money for an orphanage he and his non-profit organization, Eyes Wide Open International, were building.

The money he was withdrawing was to be used to purchase food for the orphans. As he completed his transaction in broad daylight, a group of thugs targeted him. Knowing he had withdrawn money the culprits unloaded numerous rounds in the direction of Dave at very close range while he was in his car. After hitting their target, they approached him and stole his camera and passport but neglected to take his cash, as it was stuffed deep in his pants pocket. The suspects were never found.

Dave Bompart, known lovingly as Big Dave, was a gentle giant originally from the islands of Trinidad and Tobago. He served in the military for a few years and worked with the United Nations a bit before moving to the U.S. He later met and married his wife, Nicolle. From their home city in Columbus, Ohio they created the religious-based non-profit organization Eyes Wide Open International in 2009 to provide humanitarian services internationally. Days after the earthquake, Dave packed a light bag and told his wife he was flying to Haiti to help and that was that. He showed up on the grounds of the Project Medishare Tent Hospital and asked how he could help. "He was as big as one of our tents and said can I help?" recalls Dr. Barth Green, one of the founders of Medishare. Soon he became the manager of the logistics operation and stayed with the organization for months to come. He continued to work with the hospital as it transitioned to a physical building with Hospital Bernard Mevs. Big Dave played a crucial role in the development of what we now know as Project Medishare/Hospital Bernard Mevs.

I had the honor of working with Dave numerous times. He was willing to help trouble shoot any problem and always had a smile on his face. We had a young patient in the isolation tent for confirmed tuberculosis that had lost most of his family in the earthquake. He had an older sister who was always working, leaving him alone and lonely in his isolation tent most of the day and night. The patient was in his early teen years, maybe thirteen at the time and obviously depressed. Dave and I came up with an idea: maybe a pet would help boost his morale. We discussed this in fleeting as I ran off to tend to my overburdening amount of patients; Dave took the idea and ran with it. The next day he called me to his tent and showed me what he had done. He spent the early hours of the morning making a bird cage out of scrap material. Later in the day he went out and bought a small bird to go in the cage he so cleverly created. That evening, Dave and I gave our patient the bird as a gift. Upon seeing the bird his eyes lit up as if a new flame of hope had been kindled within. Over the next few days he seemed happier and happier; the idea had worked and his mood lightened. Finally he called Dave and I back to his tent. He thanked us and said "You two and Klake (Creole for Squeak, the name he had given the bird) are my new family." That was the kind of man Big Dave was – he would think well outside of the box to help everyone and anyone he could.

After being shot and robbed, Dave knew he was blocks away from the very hospital he had helped build and walked there gripping his bleeding abdomen. Through the searing pain and smell of blood and flesh he made it to the hospital. The guards immediately recognized him and the situation and urgently let him in the gates. He underwent

*Taking Care Of Ourselves*

two operations to stabilize his bleeding. He was bleeding from the wound to the abdomen and part of his bowel had to be removed. Swollen and in critical condition, he lay in the intensive care unit fighting for his life. The same doctors, nurses, guards, and friends he had made were now his caretakers. The hospital he had helped build, the hospital which had cared for thousands of people, now cared for him.

His wounds were critical and needed a higher level of care than available in Haiti. As much as Big Dave cared for others, he often neglected himself. Without health insurance and international emergency traveler's coverage, arranging for medical evacuation (med-evac) to the United States was limited by cost. A med-evac team was ready but required payment before departure. Over the years of his humanitarian work, Dave had made thousands of friends all over the world. As soon as Nicolle heard of the tragedy, she and others began a social media fundraiser. People changed their Facebook profile pictures, made phone calls, texted and Tweeted to all their contacts. Within hours the required amount of over $40,000 was raised with more money being donated every hour. I had never seen money raised so quickly. It brought together people from all over the world that didn't know each other but did know Dave and his mission.

Nicolle flew to Haiti and helped ready Dave for the transport. She found the man she loved hooked to a ventilator and in critical condition. His eyes open, he gripped her hand as she told him she was there and wouldn't leave his side. They boarded an ambulance and were sent off on their med-evac plane. The original plan was to fly Dave back home to Columbus but during the flight he had difficulty breathing and needed a tube put into the side of his chest to drain fluid out from around the lung. He was unstable and the decision was made to fly him into Miami to the Ryder Trauma Center. There he lay connected to a ventilator and heavily sedated for eight days as doctors tried everything they could to save Big Dave. Finally, his body could take no more and on February 2, 2012, Big Dave died.

Soon after the incident, Nicolle issued a statement. She felt the act was one of desperation by people probably trying to feed their own starving families. Days after the shooting Nicolle had already forgiven the shooters, made public in a statement she released. While working in Haiti Big Dave and Nicolle adopted a teenage orphan who had lost his family in the earthquake. Dave leaves Nicolle, their son, and a daughter behind who continue his life's legacy. Eyes Wide Open continues to work on the orphanage and other humanitarian missions.

Dr. Bitar, one of two brothers who found and run Hospital Bernard Mevs and operated on Dave in Haiti said "He came to Haiti to help and he was killed in Haiti by a Haitian...it's really twisted and sad." There are risks we all knowingly take in working internationally. In a few sad instances, the risks catch up with us. Even so, we continue to go back. Nicolle once said "He would do it all over again, if it would change someone's life or bring awareness to this situation...because that's the kind of guy he is."

*Taking Care Of Ourselves*

God Bless you David and Nicolle Bompart and all the volunteers who take the risk to work in Haiti and other unfamiliar and often unstable situations elsewhere – you are true heroes.

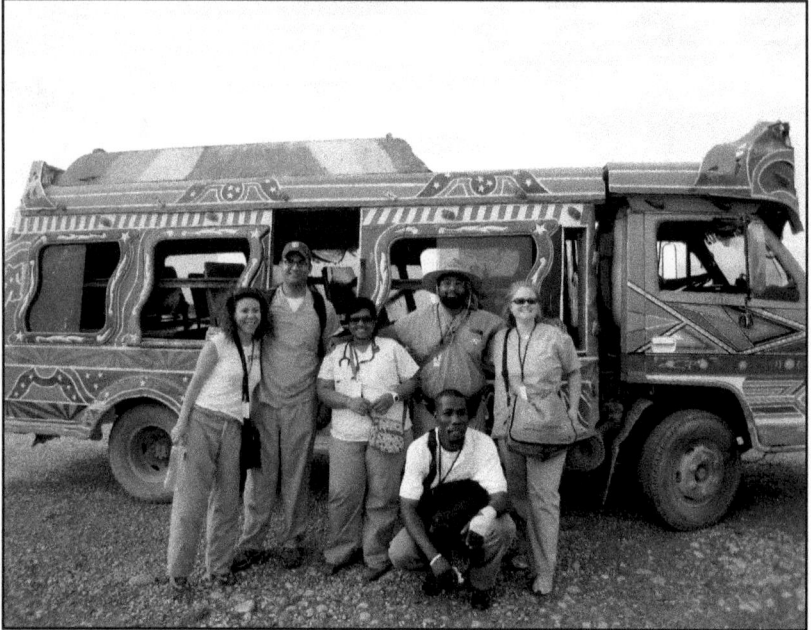

The group of us who snuck back on to the hospital grounds in a Tap Tap.

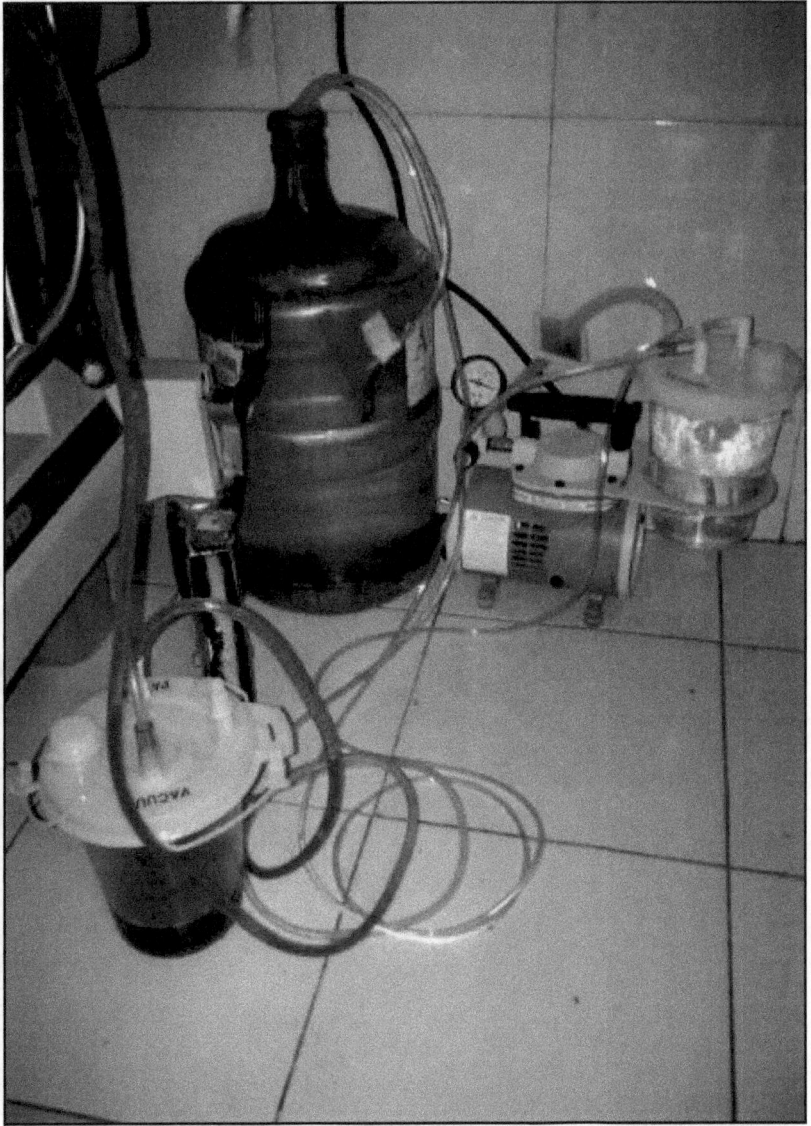

Makeshift vacuum suction rigged from a standard 5 gallon water bottle by a clever undergraduate engineering student.

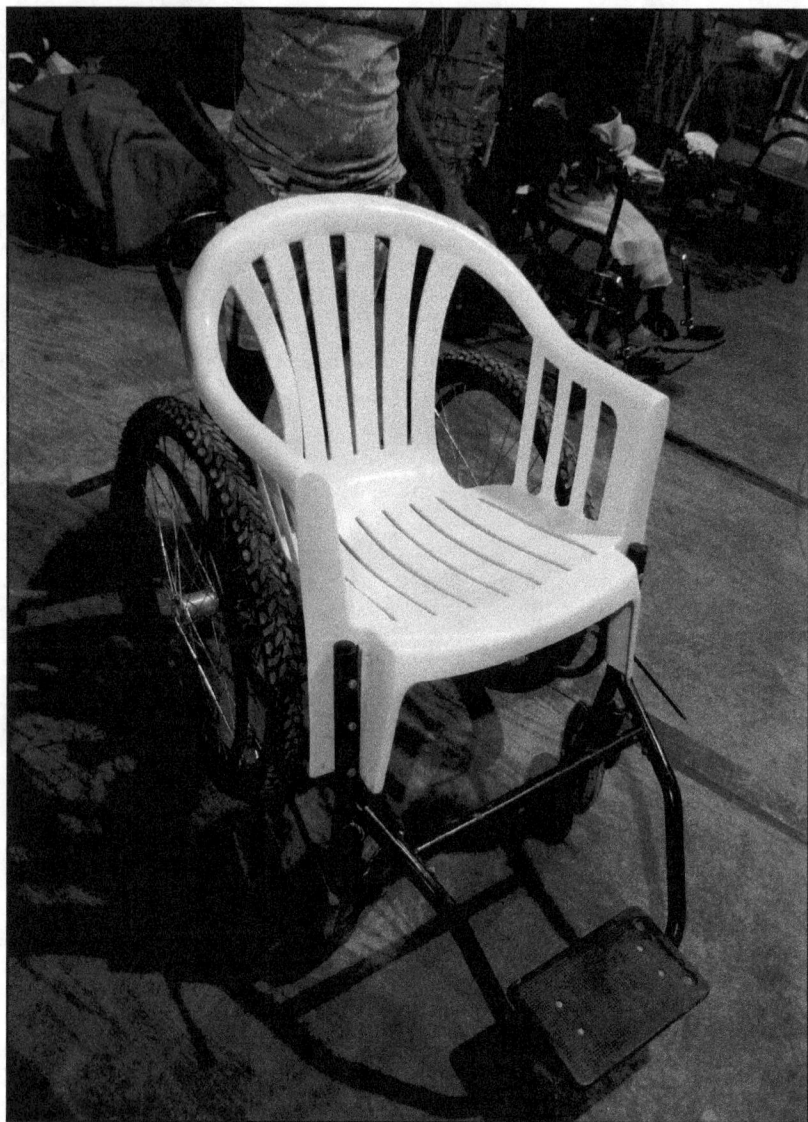

One of the many wheelchairs we used made from a basic frame
and a standard lawn chair.

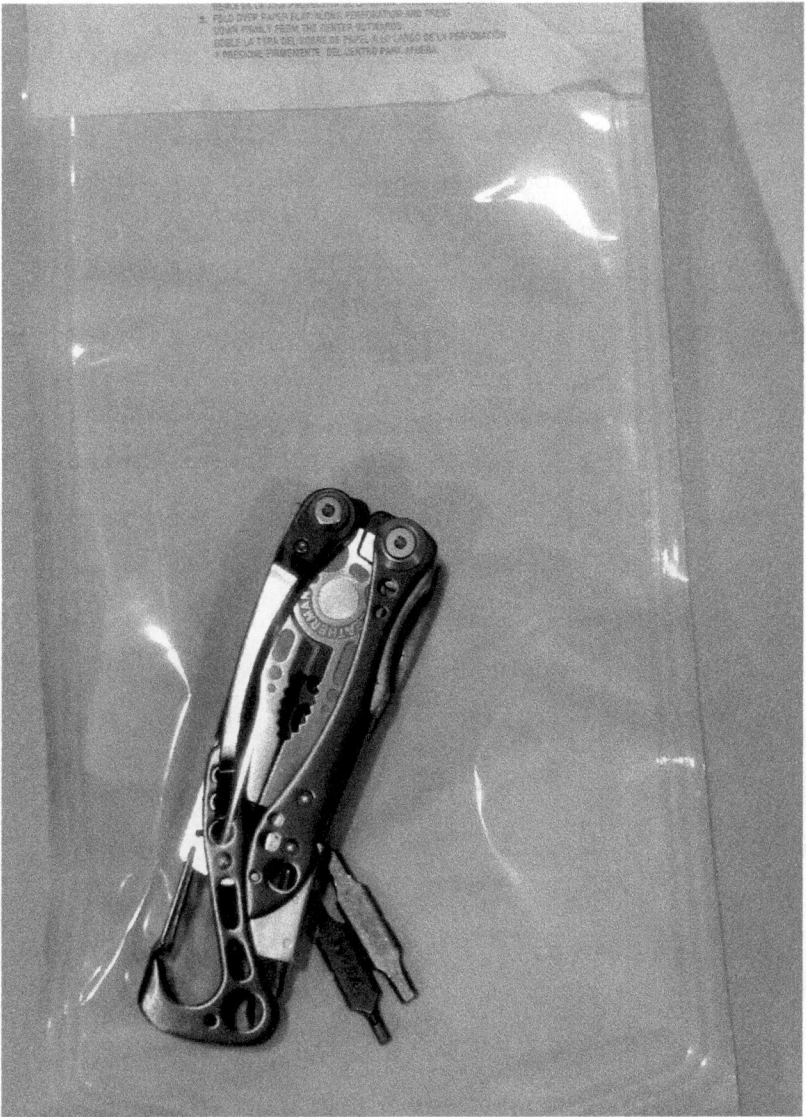

Leatherman being sterilized for use in the OR. Minimal resources meant coming up with unique solutions to unique problems.

# Closing Thoughts

Henri was a Haitian medical student who was assigned to our hospital as one of his sites of rotation. Part of our work in Haiti was to educate and work alongside our Haitian colleagues. Henri was a bit reserved – not one to be aggressive to seek out learning opportunities. He would rather wait for opportunities to find him.

A middle aged woman was wheeled into the ER complaining of difficulty breathing for weeks which had gotten worse over the past few days. Her temples were sunk and her skeletal form visible through her skin. She was emaciated. Weak and fragile, it seemed like her head was too heavy for her neck to carry. Listlessly, she moved her head back and forth as she whispered how hard it was to breathe. Given her overall sickly condition, it was obvious she either had advanced tuberculosis or HIV. Turns out she not only had HIV, but also AIDS.

AIDS is a severe syndrome in HIV where the body's white blood cell count is so low that it can't defend itself from infections from usually harmless bacteria and fungi. One of the most serious complications of AIDS is a lung infection called PCP pneumonia caused by the fungus *Pneumocystis jirovecii*. PCP pneumonia quickly eats away at the lung tissue and unless identified and treated early and aggressively, fatality is high. An x-ray of the lung confirmed my suspicion of PCP pneumonia. I asked Henri to admit her to the HIV ward and start antibiotics, steroids (to slow the inflammation and give her body a chance to fight off the infection), oxygen, and breathing treatments. The HIV ward is an isolation ward of the hospital where patients with HIV and its related complications (many of which are contagious) are admitted and treated.

Given her severity of disease on x-ray and almost corpse like physical state, I knew she didn't have long to live. Putting a breathing tube down to help her breathe was an option I had considered if she stopped breathing or had increasing difficulty with breathing. Her chance at survival either way was abysmal. At the moment, however, she was able to speak coherently and her oxygen saturation was 92%, just slightly below the cutoff for normal. Henri wheeled the patient to the HIV ward to examine her and begin his assessment. I told Henri to keep a close eye on her and have a very low threshold to come get me for help.

About fifteen minutes later Henri calmly returned and told me he needed my help. "Why," I asked. "I think she die," he replied. I ran over to the ward to find her in the wheelchair with her head limp and hanging to one side. I verified she had died and pronounced her death. Turns out Henri wheeled her over to the ward, parked her there with no nurse present, and went to go eat lunch. He came back 15 minutes later to find her sitting in a deathly pose. He did not listen to her heart or lungs or try to arouse her. Instead, he calmly walked over to me to inform me of the situation. I was shocked! Even a non-medical lay person knows the first thing to do in such a situation is to feel for a pulse or listen/look for breathing - which he had not done.

In Henri's defense, her disease was so severe she had practically no chance of survival. Yet his reaction to the situation was a bit daunting. This was not the first, nor the last time I would see this lack of urgency in Haitian medical staff. Emergencies don't rile folks up in Haiti like it does elsewhere. There was no "Code Blue" team of medical doctors, nurses, and respiratory technicians responding to start high quality cardiopulmonary resuscitation, shock the heart, put down a breathing tube, or give medications to get her heart pumping again. No constant monitoring by nurses - heck, there wasn't even a nurse in the ward to accept the patient. Who knows where she went off to or for what reason? Our resources were limited, true, but why had Henri left her without assessing her or waiting for a nurse to look after the patient? Either way she was very sick and her death was medically inevitable, but to die alone gasping for air in an empty hospital ward in the middle of the day was the tragic ending to her life's story.

Lesson learned - urgency in medicine is not a universal term, it's a cultural one. The practice of medicine in Haiti is quite different than what I am accustomed to back home. A lot stems from cultural differences. Life is slower in Haiti. Haitians tolerate much more pain and suffering and have done so longer than we have back home in the States. From their start as stolen African Slaves to the modern country of Haiti which is the poorest in the Western Hemisphere, Haitians have faced and endured suffering for hundreds of years. That doesn't mean it is any easier to lose a loved one or not be able to provide food for one's children; rather, it is expected that everyone will face some hardships during their life. One word to describe

Haitians is resilient. I thank the Haitians for imparting this valuable lesson on me.

---

I have and continue to make friends from all around the world – friends who take time off from work to leave the comfort of their home and families to help mankind half way around the world. It is humbling to say the least. The bond we share is irreplaceable and will carry on with us wherever we go.

Going to Haiti isn't cheap. Counting time taken off (mostly unpaid), medications, supplies, and airfare each trip amounts to a couple thousand dollars. Traveling to Haiti three or four times a year adds up substantially. Luckily, I have an amazing group of donors, friends, and family. Selflessly they give money, medications, supplies, and time for me to be able to make these trips. Without such support, my trips would not be possible.

Haiti is a beautiful country and Haitians are a beautiful people. Caribbean beaches, great weather, amazing food and hospitality give Haiti the potential to be a major tourist hub. Poverty, corruption, and a fragmented history of abuse and neglect, however, restrict growth. The earthquake of 2010 was just one of the many blows on the country with one major difference. The earthquake received major media coverage. For the first time in years the average American could point Haiti out on a map.

This attention was a blessing and a curse at the same time. Immediately after the earthquake it brought large amounts of financial, material, and personnel aid to the country. As time passed, however, media coverage and interest in Haiti waned. Fewer and fewer people kept up to date on the happenings of the million displaced Haitians still living in tents. Cholera, hurricanes, poverty and violence continue to batter Haiti. Rebuilding this country and bringing her up to standards of living of the 21$^{st}$ century will take decades. The only way Haiti will emerge from this nebulous state of being is to garner and maintain the interest of the international community.

Please take time to remember Haiti and do what you can to help. Volunteer your time, donate a few dollars, or even plan a trip. It's time to stop asking *Where's Haiti* and instead make your way *to* Haiti.

Orevwa e Bondye va beni nou tout! (Goodbye and God bless you all!)


~Doc Tipu

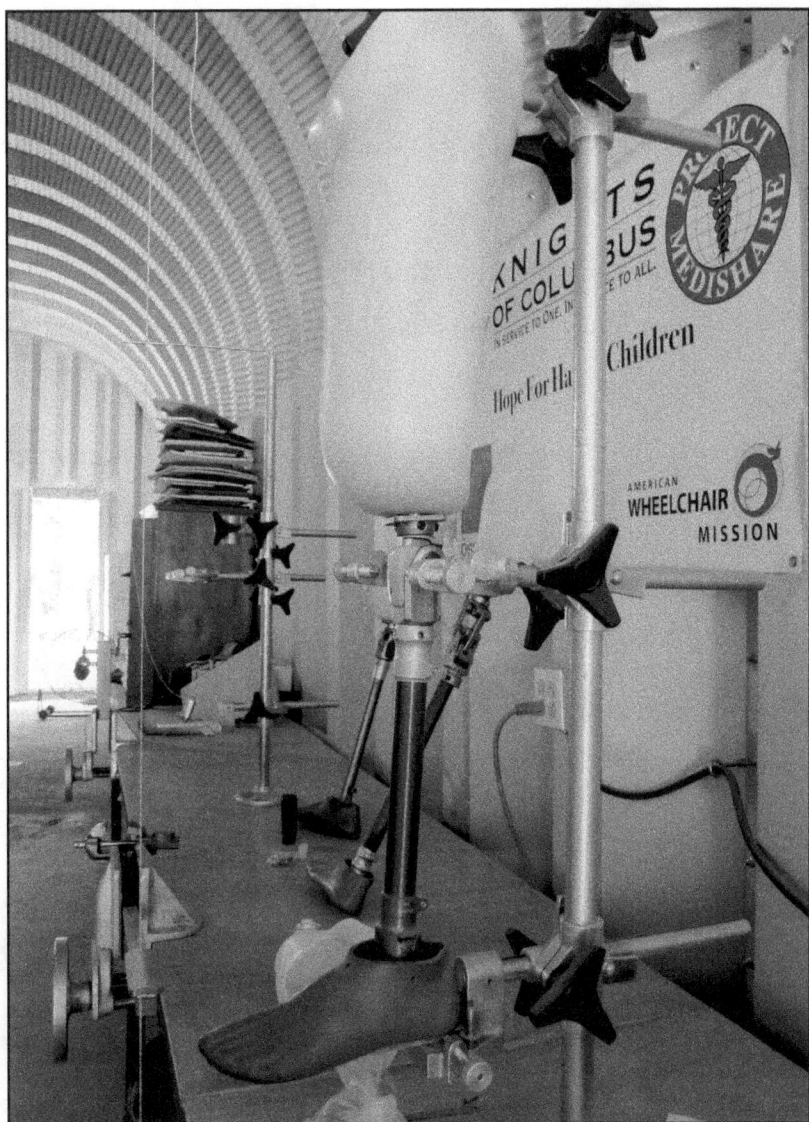

Project Medishare's prosthetics lab on the roof of the hospital.
They have fit more than 300 amputees to date.

# Acknowledgments

First and foremost I would like to thank Allah (God) for guiding me through the challenges of life.

My wife and best friend Safa. You have been my greatest support since day one. You gave me confidence and strength when I needed it the most.

My parents Tippu and Tasneem. Your sacrifice and dedication to family honed me into the man I am today.

My brother Teepu, always around to help. Without your help I would not have been able to prepare for these trips as efficiently as I did.

My extended family. We are a crazy bunch and I am thankful to have so many wonderful people in my life.

Susie Medina, my high school friend. Having you walk me through this whole process and reading my work over and over is much appreciated. Susie is an aspiring screen writer and can be followed here: www.TheFilmChild.com

Project Medishare Staff. Running a hospital is hard enough. Doing so in a disaster relief setting even more so. Thanks to all the staff who make it possible for us to come and do our jobs. www.ProjectMedishare.org

Physicians, nurses, residents, medical students, and other volunteers. We had quite a time during our trips and I remind myself how humbled I am to work with all of you. I would also like to thank all my father's colleagues. Your donations of medications and supplies were crucial during times of need.

Anthony Guarino, Seismic Analyst, California Institute of Technology for clarifying the math behind the MMS.

Drs. Theresa Nevarez, Gloria Sanchez, and Daniel Castro for working with my schedule in residency so I could make numerous trips to Haiti.

The Haitians – you are a beautiful and resilient people. Thank you for letting me come to you and do what little I could to help.

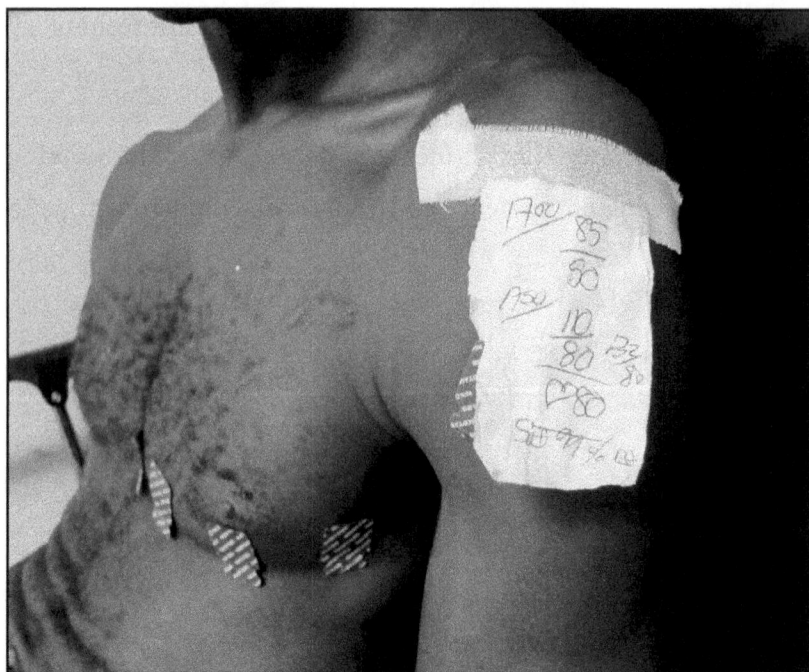

No chart, no problem. There are clever ways in Haiti to keep
track of a patient's vital signs.

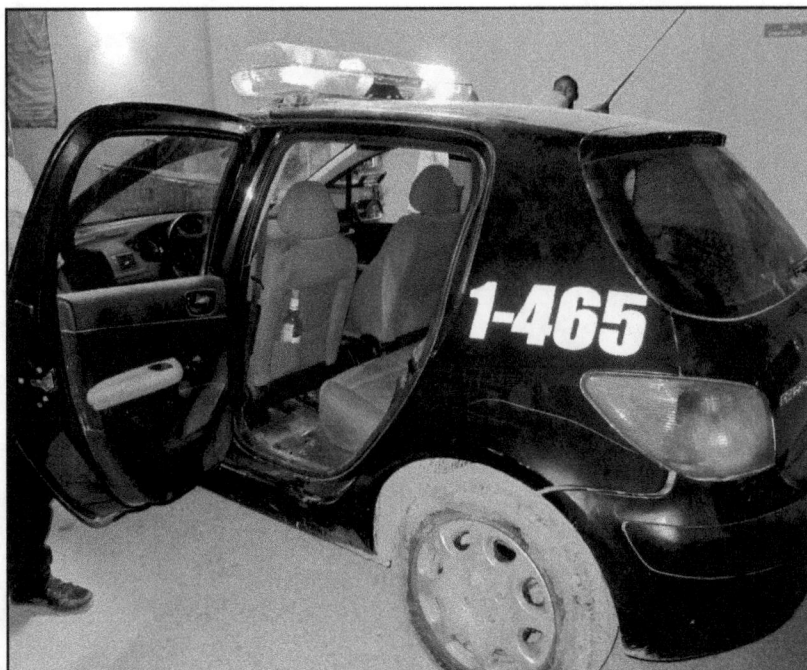

No police car in the caribbean is complete without a bottle of rum in the back

*If you have a plant in your hand and you can see the judgment day approaching, even then, without any further delay, you should sow/ put the plant in the earth.*

- Prophet Muhammad via Al-Albani -

www.ingramcontent.com/pod-product-compliance
Lightning Source LLC
Chambersburg PA
CBHW050113280326
41933CB00010B/1076